# The

# Reference

# Shelf

# Health Care

## Edited by Jennifer Peloso

The Reference Shelf
Volume 74 • Number 4

The H.W. Wilson Company
2002

# The Reference Shelf

The books in this series contain reprints of articles, excerpts from books, addresses on current issues, and studies of social trends in the United States and other countries. There are six separately bound numbers in each volume, all of which are usually published in the same calendar year. Numbers one through five are each devoted to a single subject, providing background information and discussion from various points of view and concluding with a subject index and comprehensive bibliography that lists books, pamphlets, and abstracts of additional articles on the subject. The final number of each volume is a collection of recent speeches, and it contains a cumulative speaker index. Books in the series may be purchased individually or on subscription.

Library of Congress has cataloged this serial title as follows:

Health care / edited by Jennifer Peloso.
      p.cm.—(The reference shelf; v. 74, no. 4)
      Includes bibliographical references and index.
      ISBN 0-8242-1013-1 (alk. paper)
      1. Medical care—United States. I. Peloso, Jennifer. II. Series.

RA395.A3 H3855 2002
362.1'0973—dc21

2002072732

Visit H.W. Wilson's Web site: www.hwwilson.com

Printed in the United States of America

# Contents

# *Preface*

Health care has become an extremely contentious issue throughout the United States. From college campuses to family dinner tables to executive boardrooms, Americans today are concerned with the conduct of the health care industry and the quality of health care in general. Taking their cue from the American public, Congress and the White House have engaged in heated debates over this issue. A crisis seems to be looming, due to a growing population, the approaching retirement of the baby boomer generation, and the increasing number of people who are either uninsured or insufficiently insured to meet the high costs of the care they need. Both civil service and private industry are thus trying to solve the national "ailment." The goal of this book is to present some of the many voices in the dialogue about this pressing issue and to provide a springboard from which to begin research. The emphasis is very much on health *care*—in staying healthy and treating illnesses. While not comprehensive, this collection addresses some of the most important and heavily debated aspects of health care in the United States and examines new developments in the field.

This book looks at five areas of interest in American health care today. Chapter 1 presents an overview of some of the most prevalent diseases found in the United States and profiles the top killers. These are diseases that could afflict anyone, male or female, and everyone should be aware of the risks for contracting them, their symptoms, and the approaches of the medical community towards treating them. The first article touches on topics that will be discussed in greater detail throughout the book. It briefly discusses the association between health and lifestyle, alternative medicines' role in preventing and treating disease, why insurance companies should promote healthy living, and the pharmaceutical industry's interest in the aging baby boomer generation. The next seven articles focus on a range of ailments, specifically heart disease, the nation's number-one killer, lung, prostate, and skin cancer, drug abuse, and depression. Each article discusses who is at risk for developing the disease, ways in which it may be avoided, and possible treatments.

The next chapter considers how Americans pay for their illnesses—that is, how individuals and employers bear the burden of health insurance. Over 40 million Americans are uninsured, and that number grows each year. Health insurance has therefore become one of the most heavily contested issues in the political arena, and anyone who can find a way to remedy this increasingly desperate situation will emerge as the David who defeated a Goliath. The way in which quality is sacrificed to cost in the health care system; the role of Medicare and Medicaid in the plight of the uninsured and the elderly; and the various kinds of HMOs, PPOs, and supplemental insurance policies for those with critical illnesses are examined in this chapter, "The Business of Health Care." The chapter concludes with an article addressing the current debate in Congress over a Patient's Bill of Rights, which would give people the right to sue their HMOs if they could prove negligence.

Chapters 3 and 4, "Women's Health" and "Elder Care," focus on two segments of American society whose particular health concerns have begun to receive greater attention within the medical community. For years, women were given medical advice based on research into and knowledge about the male body, despite the inherent differences in female physiology. Recently, however, women's health has emerged as an important, distinct medical field. New findings are forcing doctors to realize that women need to be examined and diagnosed differently from their male counterparts. Chapter 3 concentrates on health issues of greatest interest to women, including heart disease, breast and ovarian cancer, eating disorders, and menopause.

Chapter 4 examines the most pressing health problems facing older Americans today. These concerns do not belong exclusively to the current population of seniors, but also to their children and care givers, to the aging baby boomers who will soon reach "senior" status, and to every American citizen whose tax dollars contribute to Medicare and Medicaid—not to mention anyone who hopes to live to a "ripe old age." The articles in this chapter look at the effects of and treatments for Alzheimer's disease, the lavish array of medications being prescribed for the elderly (sometimes to the physical and mental detriment of patients), the recent suggestion that drugs can combat the effects of aging, the latest innovations in stem cell research, the impact of Medicare on the nursing home industry, and hospice care for the terminally ill.

The final chapter in the book looks at various alternatives to conventional health care that have recently gained in popularity. Disillusioned with Western medicine and frightened of its costs, many individuals have turned to alternative therapies, such as chiropractic, acupuncture, homeopathy, and herbal remedies to cure what ails them. The articles in this chapter examine the growing appeal of such treatments, along with some caveats for those thinking of using them.

I would like to thank all the authors and publications that granted permission to reprint their work. I would also especially like to thank Lynn Messina, Sandra Watson, Norris Smith and Rich Stein for their help and patience; without them, this book would not have been possible.

**Jennifer Peloso**
**August 2002**

# I. Treating Common Ailments and Diseases

# Editor's Introduction

Since ancient times, people have been plagued by diseases and ailments that they did not know how to cure. Medical advances have been made, both by diligent research and by accident. As scientists have grown in their understanding of the human body, they have been able to discover a good deal about how the body works and how it responds to certain internal and environmental conditions.

With the vast amount of knowledge available in the 21st century and the overwhelming number of drugs and medications available—not only by prescription, but also over the counter—one would think humankind would have made more progress toward curing some of the most common diseases. While we anticipate the day when some of the most fatal diseases will be merely chronic and manageable, we should also consider the words of the ancient Greek physician Hippocrates, who said that it was better to prevent a disease than to treat it. Though doctors have not yet found cures for every fatal disease, they do know ways to prevent many of them. Each person, they tell us, holds the key to good health and must accept the consequences of particular lifestyle decisions, many of which prove fatal and take lives sooner than necessary. This chapter looks at some of the most prevalent chronic illnesses and potentially fatal diseases in the United States, many of them preventable and some even curable if caught in the early stages.

The first article, "A Healthy Lifestyle," emphasizes the importance of healthy living and good nutrition in preventing diseases, including many of the maladies discussed in the rest of this chapter. It also looks at the role insurance companies could play in health maintenance, besides treating illnesses, and in the increasing role of alternative medicine.

Because more men and women in the United States die of heart disease than any other ailment, the chapter begins with an article about this condition. Once affecting only those in their later years, heart attacks now occur in 30 and 40 year olds, stressed by today's fast-paced lifestyles. Demetrios Georgiou reports on the causes of heart attacks, their symptoms, the different surgeries available to patients, drugs that can help prevent heart attacks by lowering cholesterol, and lifestyle changes that can stave off the onset of stroke or cardiac arrest.

After heart disease, the most serious threat to the health of Americans comes from cancer, still one of the most frightening and mysterious of all illnesses. The number of cancer cases in the United States is expected to rise due to a growing and aging population, according to the "Annual Report to the Nation on the Status of Cancer, 1973–1999, Featuring Implications of Age and Aging on the U.S. Cancer Burden" (*Cancer*, May 15, 2002). The next four articles in this chapter are therefore devoted to different types of cancers, which are among the most intractable of all diseases. I begin with an article by Gordon E. Katske about lung cancer, the second leading cause of natural death in both men and women. A largely preventable disease, it is usually caused by smoking or prolonged exposure to environmental factors, such as second-hand cigarette smoke, materials like asbestos, or radiation. Lung cancer results in more deaths than prostate, breast, and colon cancer combined. Prostate cancer, which is specific to males, is the second most fatal cancer among that gender, as the next article, from *Harvard Men's Health Watch,* explains. The causes of prostate cancer are currently unknown, but it is most common among African American and Hispanic men. Skin cancer, once diagnosed predominantly in those over 60, is being found today in sun worshipers as young as 20, according to the article that follows, from *Men's Fitness.* Another preventable condition, it afflicts over one million people every year, its deadliest form being melanoma. All of these articles highlight the causes, detection methods and symptoms, and treatments and/or surgeries that are available for each cancer.

Another type of illness that plagues many Americans is substance abuse, an incurable disease, according to some medical professionals. Long-term substance abuse can damage the liver, heart, brain, and nervous system. It can cause high blood pressure and stomach problems and lead to violence and fatal accidents. In the sixth article in this chapter, Joanne Wojcik discusses the limited benefits offered by employers to employees in need of substance abuse treatment. An accompanying sidebar lists those treatments recommended by the National Institution on Drug Abuse.

In the final article in this chapter, Suz Redfearn examines depression in Q&A form. Nineteen million Americans are estimated to suffer from depression, but two-thirds of those cases go untreated because they are simply missed or misdiagnosed and then treated incorrectly. Redfearn answers several important questions about this debilitating illness, including "So next time I go to the doctor, she's going to screen me for depression?"; "Will a diagnosis of depression go on my permanent medical record?"; and "If I'm diagnosed with depression, will my insurer cover treatment?"

# A Healthy Lifestyle[1]

BY PATRICK PLASKETT
*NEW TIMES NATURALLY!*, MAY–JUNE 2001

I had a man come into my office accompanied by his daughter. He was in his 50s and had recently learned that he had diabetes. His daughter thought that a hypnotist might help him modify his diet so that his condition did not get any worse. This was quite reasonable, for hypnosis is used from time to time to complement the treatment given by an allopathic practitioner of the healing arts—a medical doctor.

I asked what dietary counsel had been given by the doctor.

"None," I was told.

"None?" I asked incredulously. It was true. We as a society are so much more into disease care rather than health care that it is typical for a doctor to be trained in diagnoses of a condition and a way to medicate or otherwise treat it, and nothing more. Few medical doctors are required to take one course in nutrition to get their degree, yet few things will affect your physical health more than what you put inside your body. Fortunately for my new client, he and his daughter had done some research and had a clear idea as to what dietary habits he wanted to change. I understood this very well, and I know that, whatever a person's diet is, it is a habit in the subconscious—they can modify that habit for whatever reason.

No one needs to get a disease before sensing the need to modify a habit to ensure a long and happy life. Those people with a tendency to put on weight can change their diet and reduce the risk of cardiovascular disorder. Those people with a sedentary lifestyle can develop some regular exercise and improve the tone of the entire body. Those people that take the stress of life badly can practice relaxation techniques. Improving attitudes can improve the health. Outside of oriental medicine, it is little understood or recognized how negative attitudes have a corresponding effect on specific organs and systems of the body.

But attitudes are changing. I have a friend that has been practicing transcendental meditation for twenty years who was happy to learn that her Blue Cross insurance would cover the expense of a TM retreat that she planned to attend. I don't think that this is because Blue Cross hopes to promote meditation, but rather because they found that those who practice meditation are statisti-

---

1. Article by Patrick Plaskett from *New Times Naturally!* May/June 2001. Copyright © Altnewtimes, Inc. Reprinted with permission.

cally healthier than the general population that doesn't meditate. So, if they support the personal efforts of those insured that wish to meditate, it will save the company money in the long run.

> *The insurance companies . . . fare better when people don't get sick in the first place.*

Perhaps the real thrust of health care rather than disease care will come from the insurance companies, for they have to hand out the immediate cash every time someone requires medical attention. It is true that the number of people interested in alternative types of health therapies is at an all-time high, but I believe that this reflects a gradual word-of-mouth dissemination of natural health consciousness rather than an organized effort by anyone. Even alternative health care is often disease-oriented rather than health-oriented; someone might try acupuncture simply to make the pain go away. The insurance companies, on the other hand, fare better when people don't get sick in the first place. They stand to gain if people would adopt a healthy lifestyle.

A healthy lifestyle is really what health care is all about. Except when you are subject to some trauma like getting hit by a car, the state of your health is most likely going to be the result of your habits. Often the correlation between health and lifestyle is unclear; as an example, people can vary in sensitivity to living in a society that puts sugar in nearly all prepared food. Some people might consider diabetes a natural risk of old age, rather than a natural risk of how their particular bodies react to a lifetime of the "modern" diet. It strikes me as curious that the people who are concerned about the health of aging baby-boomers are singularly concerned with the anticipated need for drugs for chronic conditions rather than anything that would keep the aging population healthy. Perhaps it is politically incorrect to suggest anything that would interfere with the flow of money into the health-care system.

What can you do for your personal health care? Adopt a healthy lifestyle! But what is that? That could depend on who you talk to. My advice is to listen to everyone who has any knowledge on the subject. Read books and magazine articles, too. Examine what your present habits are, and choose one to improve. What do you eat? What thoughts do you entertain all day long? Impressions are food too. How do you exercise? How do you handle stress? All of these things are under your control, and can affect your health. There will always be a need for the physician that can handle trauma such as a broken leg or sew up a gash. There will always be a need for a surgeon who can cut out a tumor. But there is always room for improvement in our knowledge of what a healthy lifestyle is, and room for improvement in our habits of implementing what we know to be good and worthwhile.

# Heart Attack! Prevention and Treatment[2]

By Demetrios Georgiou
*USA Today Magazine*, July 2001

Often, you hear people say that an individual seemed perfectly healthy, but suddenly died from a heart attack. In the past, cardiac specialists assumed that a person's chance of having a heart attack is higher if there are severe blockages in the coronary artery, and the larger the blockage, the greater the risk. The more severe blockages often will cause symptoms of chest pain (angina) because the heart does not get enough blood, especially when the patient exerts himself or herself. Consequently, common sense would dictate that most people who develop heart attacks must have severe blockages.

However, over the past 10 years, results of scientific studies defied common sense and showed that, in fact, the most dangerous blockages are often not the largest. This new knowledge came from studies where patients who had a heart attack underwent angiography (an X-ray of the heart and blood vessels following a dye injection) to determine the magnitude of the blockage (stenosis) in the vessel prior to the heart attack. The average stenosis was about 50% of the diameter of the coronary artery. The more severe blockages—a 70% stenosis or greater—were often not the cause of the heart attack. In view of these findings, the question arises: If heart attacks are caused by an obstruction of blood flow to the heart, how can smaller blockages be more dangerous than larger ones? Furthermore, if severe narrowing of an artery is not the cause of a heart attack, what is?

The nature of the plaques that make up the blockages turns out to be the key in the development of a heart attack. The plaques contain a mix of cholesterol, fats, fibrous tissue, and white blood cells that deposit in the walls of the arteries over time. There is a great variability in plaque composition. Studies found that plaques that contain a lot of cholesterol and less cells (less fibrous tissue)—the so-called "soft" or unstable plaques—are more likely to rapture and cause a heart attack. The plaques that contain very little cholesterol and more cells are called "hard" or stable plaques and are less likely to rupture and, thus, less likely to cause a heart attack.

2.  Article by Demetrios Georgiou, M.D., from *USA Today* July 2001. Copyright © Society for the Advancement of Education. Reprinted with permission.

---

# Heart Disease and Stroke Still Leading Killers

Heart disease and stroke are the first and third leading causes of death for both men and women among all groups in the United States. They are also major causes of disability. Although cardiovascular disease is often thought to affect mostly men and older people, it is a major killer of women and people in the prime of life.

More than 60 million Americans have some form of cardiovascular disease, including high blood pressure, coronary heart disease, stroke, congestive heart failure and other conditions.

More than 2,600 Americans die each day of cardiovascular disease. That is an average of one death every 33 seconds.

The economic impact of cardiovascular disease on the health care system continues to grow as the population ages, reaching $299 billion in 2001.

Three health-related behaviors contribute markedly to the problem:

- Tobacco use. Smokers have twice the risk for heart attack as nonsmokers. Nearly one-fifth of all deaths from cardiovascular disease, or about 190,000 deaths a year, are smoking-related.

- Lack of physical activity. People who are sedentary are twice as likely to get heart disease than people who are active. More than half of adults do not exercise enough.

- Poor nutrition. People who are overweight have a higher risk for cardiovascular disease. Only 18 percent of women and 20 percent of men report eating five servings of fruits and vegetables each day. Almost 60 percent of U.S. adults are overweight or obese.

Modifying these behaviors is critical both for preventing and controlling cardiovascular disease.

## The Risk Factors

Individual factors that put people at increased risk for cardiovascular diseases include:

- High blood pressure
- High blood cholesterol
- Tobacco use
- Physical inactivity
- Poor nutrition
- Overweight obesity
- Diabetes

*Source:* Article from *State Legislatures* February 2002. Copyright © National Conference of State Legislatures. Reprinted with permission.

---

One might ask what triggers the plaque rupture because, if we know the reason(s) that precipitate it, we would be able to take measures to prevent a rupture and, thus, the heart attack.

There is a hot debate in the scientific community about the factors that trigger the rupture of plaque, but, to date, we do not know the reasons. One thing is certain: The stable plaques are characterized by a predominantly hard fibrous tissue with a thick covering, called fibrous cap, as strong as the ligaments in your knee. These types of plaques contain very little cholesterol and grow very slowly over the years. The heart has its own ways to deal with the blockages when blood flow is decreased in certain areas of the heart muscle. So, just as if a major freeway to a city is closed and commuters find side streets to get to town, the heart similarly tries to develop smaller, new arteries to feed the area of the muscle in need, called collateral vessels. These collateral vessels act as a natural bypass to the clogged artery and bring the necessary blood and oxygen to the heart muscle in jeopardy. This is a very important way the heart has to resolve the problem of shortage in blood supply flowing to the area in need. Stable plaques are rarely responsible for a heart attack. Even if, in some patients, arteries become completely blocked, the heart muscle remains healthy because the heart had time to grow collateral arteries.

On the other hand, the unstable plaque, characterized by a large lipid pool and a very thin cover, will rupture suddenly and cause a heart attack because the heart did not have the time to grow collateral vessels. The thin cap ruptures easily, and a blood clot is formed quickly and sits on top of the ruptured plaque, causing severe blockage, cutting the nutrients and oxygen to the heart muscle. Depending on the size of the area involved, one can have a small or a large heart attack.

*Studies have demonstrated that patients with heart attacks can benefit significantly from exercise training.*

Say two people have a heart attack, and one survives while the other dies suddenly before he or she was able to reach the hospital. In the first case, the patient lived because he or she had collateral circulation substituting for the blocked vessel. In the second instance, the patient died because he or she did not have the collateral circulation to supply the heart muscle in need with oxygen and other nutrients. The muscle dies, and electrical instability takes place in the form of a chaotic rhythm that is very rapid, called ventricular fibrillation. With this chaotic rhythm, the patient cannot sustain a blood pressure, and death follows.

It is of critical importance to have collateral vessels in place because their absence or presence may be a matter of life and death. Studies have demonstrated that patients with heart attacks can benefit significantly from exercise training. After eight weeks of bicycling on a stationary bike three times a week for 30-40 minutes, subjects were able to grow new vessels which helped improve the blood supply to the area of the heart attack by about 30%. This is very good news for heart attack victims. It is vital to emphasize, though, that before anybody engages in any physical activity, that individual should first visit his or her physician to make sure that there is no danger in doing so. The initial stage of workouts (first eight weeks) should be supervised by trained personnel.

People who develop symptoms of chest pain should seek medical attention immediately. Everyone, including those who never had any symptoms of chest pain, must understand what the early signs of a heart attack are. The American Heart Association recommends that people call 911 or the local emergency number immediately if they experience any of the following symptoms:

- Uncomfortable pressure, fullness, squeezing, or pain in the center of the chest lasting more than a few minutes
- Pain spreading to the shoulders, neck, or arms
- Chest discomfort with lightheadedness, fainting, sweating, nausea, or shortness of breath.

If you are having a heart attack, time is against you. Today, there are very good medications to dissolve the clots that cause a heart attack. Therefore, if you get to the emergency room within, say, two hours from the onset of chest pain, doctors can treat you and save a significant amount of heart muscle, thus aborting a heart attack. The message is: Get to the Emergency Room early. The earlier you do, the better your chances will be.

Once a heart attack takes place, there are excellent medications to help patients. The alternatives are catheter therapies with balloon angioplasty and stents—metallic devices to open the artery—and bypass (open heart) surgery, where the surgeon uses veins and arteries from the arms and/or legs to bypass the blockages.

> *Get to the Emergency Room early. The earlier you do, the better your chances will be.*

None of these solutions are curative. Even after a successful procedure, the arteries may reocclude (close up), a phenomenon called restenosis. The rate of restenosis can range from 12 to 50%, depending on the type of procedure performed. There is a lot of research going on to try to tackle this problem, but results so far have been disappointing. In deciding which approach to take, catheter intervention is less traumatic and you can recover and go back to work faster. However, because of the restenosis problem, you should be prepared to return to the hospital for multiple catheter procedures. If, on the other hand, you elect to have bypass surgery, it is more traumatic and will take you longer to recover fully, but you will not need to repeat the procedure as often.

Hippocrates, the father of modem medicine, said that it is better to prevent a disease than to treat it. This statement was true in the fifth century and still is today. Given the problem of restenosis and the inability to cure coronary artery disease, prevention certainly makes a lot of sense. Realistically speaking, though, while coronary artery disease cannot be prevented completely, a great deal can be done to reduce its risk. Lifestyle changes become very important to achieve this goal, and need to be underscored in every case with coronary artery disease.

Doctors as well as patients tend to focus on coronary artery disease in an individual's 60s and 70s, when it often is too late, since the condition is fully developed or a heart attack has taken place.

Rather, focus needs to be on the 30s and 40s, when there is time to make appropriate changes and reduce the chance of a heart attack. Seek medical attention when you are well. Visit your heart specialist regularly and have a stress test. Physicians can diagnose coronary artery disease by doing a stress test, so that, if a problem is detected, it can be taken care of on time, before a heart attack takes place.

Unfortunately for some of their patients, many doctors focus more on mechanical procedures, rather than on controlling blood sugar, lowering cholesterol, diet, smoking cessation, and exercise training. As a result, the patient will either have a reocclusion or a heart attack. Lifestyle modifications may be more important than the catheter procedures.

Many studies have shown that medications called statins that lower cholesterol—such as Zocor, Lipitor, and Pravachol, just to mention a few—will reduce the fat content and increase the stability of plaques. Epidemiological studies have shown that, for each one percent reduction in cholesterol level, there is a two percent lowering in the risk of a heart attack. More recent studies with the newer statins have shown even more striking benefits: on average, a 20–30% reduction in heart attacks in people with or without coronary artery disease, but with high levels of cholesterol and other risk factors. The statins are safe and side effects—such as inflammation of the liver (hepatitis) and inflammation of the muscles (myositis)—are rare. Overall, they are safer than aspirin, which can cause stomach bleeding. You should visit your doctor to determine your risk for a heart attack and whether or not you should be taking cholesterol-lowering medications.

**A healthy diet.** Along with regular exercise, a healthy diet is one of the most important things you can do to affect your overall health positively. Reducing fat in your diet, for example, can lower your risk for certain cancers and coronary artery disease.

Eat plenty of vegetables and fish, as well as cook with olive oil. It is important to eat a balanced diet. That means 30% of your diet should contain fat, 30% carbohydrates, and 40% protein. There is a lot of emphasis on the Mediterranean diet because coronary artery disease is less common in those countries than in the U.S. The basis of the Mediterranean diet is olive oil, fresh fruits, and vegetables.

**Exercise training.** Talk to your physician about a regular exercise program. Aerobic exercises such as walking, swimming, or bicycling can help condition your heart and improve circulation. Begin slowly; increase your workload gradually; and see your doctor if you experience any discomfort while exercising.

Scientific studies have shown clearly that if you have had a heart attack and you exercise two or three times a week for 30-40 minutes, not only can you improve your exercise capacity, but your heart will develop collaterals that will improve the circulation in the area of the heart attack. In other words, your heart is capable of regrowing smaller arteries, which act like a natural bypass. In addition, the weakened heart muscle becomes stronger after the heart attack. Before you engage in any physical activity, you should speak to your doctor and have a stress test done.

**Quit smoking.** Smoking can aggravate angina and may have harmful effects on your heart arteries. The nicotine contained in the cigarettes destroys the inner layer of the arteries called endothelium, which, in turn, will cause plaque to form and grow more rapidly and ultimately lead to a heart attack or stroke.

**Take your medication.** Always take your medication according to your physician's instructions. Remember to do so at the same time every day. One of the reasons doctors have difficulties controlling high blood pressure is patients' poor compliance with their medications.

With an aging population, cardiovascular disease is likely to remain the number-one killer in this country. Coronary artery disease is a chronic process causing a lot of physical and, in some cases, mental disability. Despite advances in treatment, coronary artery disease still has no cure. The best strategy remains risk factor modification and changes in lifestyle.

# Early Detection One Key to Stopping Lung Cancer[3]

By Gordon E. Katske
*BUSINESS JOURNAL*, JULY 14, 2000

Primary llung cancer remains the leading cause of death from malignancy for men and women in the United States.

This year, an estimated 164,100 new cases will be diagnosed in this country. Sadly, about 156,900 patients will die from the disease in the same period.

Lung cancer causes more deaths than the combined mortality from colon, breast, and prostate cancers. The five-year combined survival rate for all stages of lung cancer was 14 percent in 1995, the last year for which national data is available.

Most cases of lung cancer are discovered between the ages of 50 and 60.

Of all cases, 56 percent occur in men. If lung cancer is detected before it has spread to the lymph nodes or other organs, the five-year survival rate is about 42 percent with aggressive surgical treatment. Unfortunately, only one-fifth of all lung cancer cases are detected at an early stage.

Cigarette smoking causes 80 percent of lung cancer cases. The longer a person smokes cigarettes, the greater the chance of developing lung cancer. The smoker also adversely affects the health of the people around him. Non-smoking spouses of smokers have a 30 percent greater risk of developing lung cancer than do spouses of nonsmokers.

Non-smoking workers exposed to tobacco smoke in the workplace are also more likely to develop lung cancer.

Exposure to asbestos and radon gas in the work place also increases the risk of developing lung cancer. These exposures are amplified if the worker smokes or is exposed to secondhand smoke.

Patients who have had lung cancer in the past are at greater risk of developing a second new lung cancer. Age also plays an important role in the development of lung cancer. Recent research suggests that the lung cells of the elderly are more likely to develop a malignancy, when exposed to cigarette smoke, than are lung cells of younger patients.

---

Cigar and pipe smoking cause lung cancer at almost the same rate as cigarette smoking. There is no evidence that smoking low tar or nicotine cigarettes reduces the risk of developing lung cancer.

Contrary to popular opinion, air pollution is not a major cause of lung cancer. Many studies have proved that air pollution only slightly increases the risk of developing lung cancer. This risk is dwarfed by the enormous hazard imposed by all forms of tobacco use.

Early detection and aggressive surgical treatment are the keys to long-term survival and cure. Patients must be on the alert for the signs and symptoms of lung cancer. A persistent cough, wheezing or hoarseness together with shortness of breath and unexplained weight loss are symptoms of concern.

Chest pain, recurrent bronchitis or coughing up blood should also be a reason to seek medical care.

The detection of lung cancer begins with a complete history and physical exam performed by a doctor. A chest X-ray and a CT scan are the most important imagining tests to localize a lung tumor. Looking into the patient's lungs with a bronchoscope and taking

---

### *Early detection and aggressive surgical treatment are the keys to long-term survival and cure.*

---

biopsies is the most frequent technique for establishing the diagnosis of lung cancer.

A board certified thoracic surgeon with special training in cancer surgery should direct the surgical care of the patient with lung cancer.

This specialist must be ready and able to apply the latest and most advanced techniques to the care of the patient.

When lung cancer is diagnosed, an attempt must be made to rule out spread of the disease to other parts of the body. Sampling the lymph nodes of the chest and performing CT scans of the abdomen and bone scans gives a clear picture of the extent of the disease and helps determine the best treatment.

There are basically two forms of lung cancer: small-cell and non-small-cell.

Small-cell lung cancer accounts for about 20 percent of all lung cancers. This type of cancer contains cells that are small and that multiply quickly, spreading to other area of the body like the lymph nodes, the brain, the liver, and the bones in the early stages of the disease.

The diagnosis of this tumor is established surgically but it is most often treated with a combination of chemotherapy and radiation

Small cell lung cancer is usually caused by smoking. Non-small cell lung cancer is the most common type of lung cancer, accounting for almost 80 percent cases. This type of cancer is slower growing and spreads to other parts of the body later. This form of lung cancer is usually diagnosed and treated with surgery, sometimes in conjunction with chemotherapy and radiation.

Non-small cell lung cancer is also usually caused by smoking.

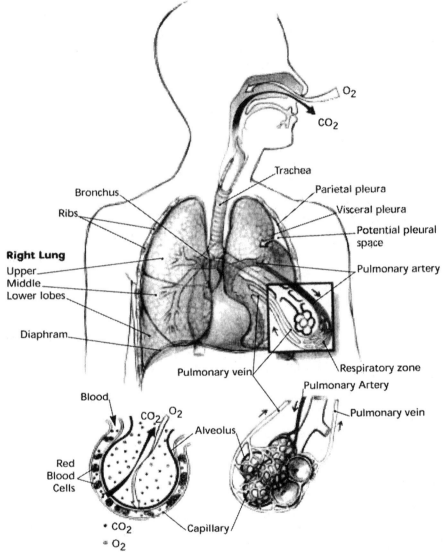

**Lung Structure and Respiration**

Inhaled air travels through the airways to the alveoli. Blood is pumped out of the heart through the pulmonary arteries to a network of capillaries that surround the alveoli. The oxygen of the inhaled air diffuses out of the alveoli into the blood while carbon dioxide in the blood moves into the alveoli to be exhaled. The oxygen-rich blood is returned to the heart through the pulmonary veins.

*Source:* National Heart, Lung, and Blood Institute, *www.nhlbi.nih.gov*

# Prostate Cancer: Three Research Advances[4]

*HARVARD MEN'S HEALTH WATCH*, JUNE 2002

Scientists have made important progress in understanding the biology of prostate cancer, and clinicians are increasingly able to use that information to improve diagnosis and treatment. But prostate cancer is like a jigsaw puzzle: The outlines may be clear, but many pieces are still out of place. Still, it's nice to know that scientists continue to make advances; for example, recent studies have produced findings in three different areas that may help find a solution to the prostate cancer puzzle.

## Epidemiology

Who gets prostate cancer? Any man can, but some men are at higher risk than others. For example, men who live in the U.S. are more vulnerable than their Asian peers, and in America itself, risk is distributed unequally. For years, doctors have known that African Americans are more likely to die from prostate cancer (4% risk) than whites (3%). A new study reveals that Hispanics are also at greater risk. In addition, the research helps account for the racial disparities. In the case of Hispanics, the increased risk can be explained entirely by socioeconomic (income, education, and access to medical care) and lifestyle (dietary) factors. But while these factors contribute to the prostate cancer problem in blacks, they don't tell the whole story. Instead, genetics, hormones, or other biologic elements add to the risk. It's an important area for future research.

## Etiology

What causes prostate cancer? It's the $64,000 question, but doctors don't know the answer—yet. Still, a recent study may help by confirming a 1996 Harvard report implicating insulin-like growth factor-I (IGF-I) in the disease.

IGF-I is a hormone produced by many organs such as the liver and, to a lesser degree, the prostate. IGF-I is essential for normal cell growth, but excessive levels might lead to excessive cell growth, including the growth of cancer.

The original Harvard study reported that men with the highest IGF-I levels were 4.3 times more likely to develop prostate cancer than men with the lowest levels. The newer research from Sweden confirmed an association between rising levels of IGF-I and an

---

4. Excerpted from the June 2002 issue of the *Harvard Men's Health Watch*, © 2002, President and Fellows of Harvard College.

increased risk of prostate cancer. It's intriguing work, but finding an association between two events does not prove that one causes the other—nor does it show if a treatment that reduces IGF-I can protect against prostate cancer. More questions for scientists to investigate.

**Treatment Targets**

When it comes to treating prostate cancer, doctors have many tools at their disposal. They can treat (and often cure) early disease with surgery or radiation, and they can treat (and usually control) advanced disease with radiation or by depriving the cells of androgens, the male hormones that drive the growth of prostate cells. Unfortunately, prostate cancer can escape from the effects of androgen deprivation. New research raises the possibility that a different approach may help. It's still only a gleam in the eye, but when it comes to advanced prostate cancer, any reasonable possibility warrants study.

The new potential treatment target is a gene called HER-2. It's new for prostate cancer, but it's a well-established factor in breast cancer. Excessive HER-2 activity contributes to about 25% of all breast cancers, and an antibody called trastuzumab can help in these cases. In fact, the FDA has approved the drug, which is available commercially as Herceptin.

Earlier studies of HER-2 and prostate cancer have produced contradictory and confusing findings, with reports of HER-2 activity in prostate cancer ranging from 0 to 100. But the new research may help explain the contradiction. It found that HER-2 is more active in advanced disease than in early cases, particularly in tumors that have escaped androgen deprivation therapy. It's far too early to know if treatment that targets HER-2 will help; in fact, the first trial of Herceptin has been disappointing. But men who have escaped androgen deprivation therapy are just the ones who need help the most, and scientists are sure to continue exploring treatments that aim at HER-2 as well as other targets still unknown. Stay tuned.

# Skin Cancer Casts a Giant Shadow[5]

*MEN'S FITNESS*, JUNE 2002

Sun damage doesn't just turn your skin into leather saddlebags. It can be downright deadly.

More than a million Americans each year are affected by one of the three types of skin cancer: basal cell carcinoma (the most common of all cancers), squamous cell carcinoma, or melanoma. During the past 10 years, the number of new cases of melanoma, the most dangerous form of skin cancer, has increased more rapidly than that of any other cancer. The average patient has also gotten much younger. In 1980, skin cancers were mostly found at age 60 and over. Today, patients are being diagnosed in their 20s.

Skin cancer generally occurs on the face, ears, neck, scalp, shoulders and back. People with fair hair, blue or green eyes and light complexions are most at risk, but dark-skinned people can be affected as well, sometimes on the palms or soles, in the mouth or rectum, or under fingernails or toenails. Although the vast majority of skin cancers are caused by overexposure to the sun, they can also show up on the sites of burns, scars, tattoos, contact with arsenic or radiation, or inflammatory skin conditions such as psoriasis.

Having a large number of moles seems to be a risk factor. See a doctor if any mole changes size, thickness or color. Moles that itch, hurt, bleed, ooze or scab are also suspicious. Have any mole that appeared after age 21 checked out.

## It's All Done with Mirrors

Find skin cancer in its earliest stages—while it's confined to the top layers of the skin—and it's 100 percent curable. And since the vast majority of cancers can be recognized with the naked eye, usually appearing as a blemish or altered mole, it's advisable to perform a self-check every three months. If you've already been treated for any kind of skin cancer, see your dermatologist quarterly and perform the mirror exam monthly.

## Skin Cancer ABCs and Ds

**Asymmetry:** Melanomas and other skin cancers usually have irregular shapes.

---

---

### Sunday School: How to Protect Yourself

1. Don't sunbathe.

2. Avoid unnecessary sun exposure, especially between 10 a.m. and 4 p.m., the peak hours for harmful ultraviolet radiation.

3. Sunscreen use can prevent skin cancer. Choose products rated SPF 15 or higher that block both UVA and UVB rays. And don't be stingy: Coat yourself with about one teaspoon for the face and neck and one to three tablespoons for the body (depending on how brief your briefs are). Apply 30 minutes before sun exposure and reapply frequently. Oil-free sunscreen sprays can be used on the scalp.

4. Wear protective clothing, such as long pants, long-sleeved shirts, broadbrimmed, closely woven hats and UV-protective sunglasses. Some cottons and other summer fabrics only offer SPFs of 5 to 9; light, loosely fitting synthetic fabrics with a tight weave offer the most protection.

5. Avoid artificial tanning devices. They are as dangerous as the sun, perhaps more so.

6. Take added precautions when you're on snow or water. The reflected glare nearly doubles the UV danger.

7. If you're at high risk, consider adding ultraviolet-blocking films, such as Llumar UV Shield or Vista Window Film, to your house and car windows.

8. Preliminary research indicates that antioxidants may protect against skin cancer. Make sure you get at least the recommended Daily Value of vitamins C (60 mg) and E (30 IU) and the beta-carotene in vitamin A (5,000 IU).

---

**Border:** They often have ragged and poorly defined edges or rolled borders.

**Color:** They can be very dark, multicolored or mottled with shades of black, brown and tan, or even white, gray, red or blue. Basal cell cancer can be indicated by pink growths or pale, yellow or waxy scarlike areas.

**Diameter:** They may be larger than a quarter-inch (the size of an eraser tip). Basal cell can appear as larger reddish patches, which may crust, itch or hurt.

To perform a self-exam, start with your face and scalp. Pay close attention to your nose, lips, mouth and ears; use a hand mirror to examine the backs of your ears and your scalp. (If you have thick hair, a blow-dryer can clear a visible path; ask a friend or family member to help you.)

Check your hands thoroughly, including under your nails and between your fingers, and work up toward your shoulders. Use a full-length mirror to see the sides of your upper arms, elbows and underarms.

## Not Quite Cancer

Certain conditions are associated with the eventual development of squamous cell carcinoma, according to the Skin Cancer Foundation. They include:

- Actinic keratoses: These are rough, scaly, slightly raised growths that range in color from brown to red and may be up to once inch in diameter.
- Actinic cheilitis: A type of actinic keratosis that occurs on the lips (usually the lower lip), it causes the skin to become dry, cracked, scaly, and pale or white.
- Leukoplakia: This condition is marked by white patches on the tongue or inside the mouth.
- Bowen's disease: This is a superficial squamous cell cancer that hasn't yet spread. It appears as a persistent red-brown, scaly patch, which may resemble psoriasis or eczema.

Next, examine the front of your neck, chest and torso. Finish your upper body using the hand mirror and the full-length mirror. Start with the back of your neck, then the backs of your shoulders and upper arms and continue down to your lower back.

Using both mirrors, inspect your buttocks and the backs of your legs. Sit down to inspect your feet, including under the toenails, between the toes, and the soles. Move up the ankles, shins, thighs, and sides of both legs.

Finally, since skin cancer can appear in those keep-it-covered places, examine your genital area using the hand mirror.

## Bid Bye-Bye to Baby Oil

Even if you emerge unblemished from your skin check, it's probably time to retire your cocoa-buttered weekends at the beach. Skin cancer can appear years after the sun does its work.

Other sun damage is just as sneaky. In a study at Iowa State University, three-quarters of the college-age subjects showed signs of sun damage, and more than half that group had extreme damage. However, sun habits didn't change until investigators took special UV-filter photographs to convince the students that they were risking their health as well as speeding up the skin-aging process.

True colors, indeed.

# Adapting Benefit Plans to Fit New Detox Programs[6]

By Joanne Wojcik
*Business Insurance*, July 31, 2000

In the recent film "28 Days," actress Sandra Bullock plays a hip New York socialite whose habitual partying lands her in a 28-day inpatient detoxification program.

Although this modern look at life in rehab may have looked good on the big screen, such residential alcohol treatment programs are fast disappearing.

Today, rehab providers are finding that the old-fashioned 28-day inpatient program, which was once the standard treatment for drug and alcohol abuse, doesn't work for everyone, and, in fact, often leads to relapse.

Instead, they now mold treatment to the individual, usually combining shorter, three-to five-day, inpatient detoxification programs with intensive outpatient therapy.

But not all benefit plans are keeping pace with this evolution in chemical dependency treatment, behavioral health experts point out. In fact, many employers are cutting back on the availability of treatment alternatives, either by limiting benefits to inpatient detox programs or by capping the number of times an employee can use the benefit during his or her lifetime.

The origin of the 28-day treatment program is a mystery to many in the field, even though it was the standard of treatment for years.

While some say it developed according to the level of coverage that was provided under the benefit plans of most insured employees, it actually was based on the clinical treatment of chronic male alcoholics in the late 1950s at a state hospital in Minnesota, according to Ron Hunsicker, president and chief executive officer of the National Assn. of Addiction Treatment Providers in Lititz, Pa.

"For whatever reason, the Blue Cross/Blue Shield plans picked up on that, and it became the standard benefit in health plans," he explained.

"It made sense at the time," Mr. Hunsicker said. But, since then, "most of us have long since decided that's not the standard. The one-size-fits-all approach doesn't work."

---

6. Reprinted with permission from *Business Insurance*. Issue of July 31, 2000, copyright 2000. Crain Communications Inc. All rights reserved.

Furthermore, any program that treats alcohol or drug addiction as an event, rather than as a chronic condition, will be unsuccessful, he said.

"An alcoholic or someone addicted to other drugs is never cured," he said. "It's a lifelong, chronic disease. Therefore, they need ongoing treatment, just as if they had diabetes, hypertension or asthma."

Managed care companies were perhaps among the first to recognize this, instituting chemical dependency programs that focus more on ongoing outpatient treatment than on acute inpatient care, said Pamela Greenberg, executive director of the American Managed Behavioral Healthcare Assn. in Washington.

"This is one of the things managed care has brought to the table. Other settings are considered, and treatment decisions are made on an individual basis, rather than having insurance benefits dictate the treatment level," Ms. Greenberg said.

Unfortunately, "there are situations where tailored treatment may not be covered, which is why we support mental health parity," she said.

---

### *"[Addicts] need ongoing treatment, just as if they had diabetes, hypertension or asthma."*—Ron Hunsicker, National Assn. of Addiction Treatment Providers

---

When Congress passed the Mental Health Parity Act, it did not apply to chemical dependency treatment benefits. This is because inpatient detox treatment is covered under the medical portion of most benefit plans.

But since parity was enacted, many employers have cut benefits for chemical dependency treatment while modifying mental health benefit packages.

Chicago-based Hartmarx Corp., for example, now limits the number of times its plan will cover detoxification to twice per lifetime, according to Mike Pikelny, benefits actuary.

This is a pretty common limit, according to Dr. David Whitehouse, corporate medical director at CIGNA Behavioral Health in Minneapolis.

"Most benefits for substance abuse are employer-specific, with large employers offering better benefits. Small employers have a much more punitive attitude. They say they can't afford to employ substance abusers, so we see a lot of two (per) lifetime detox benefits," he said.

"But this is completely inappropriate, because substance abuse is a relapsing illness," he said. Dr. Whitehouse also regards addiction as a chronic illness that requires regular attention. "It also drives people underground," so that they don't seek treatment when they need it, he said.

In fact, Dr. Whitehouse said that, based on CIGNA's experience, 50% of people who seek treatment for depression also have substance abuse problems, and these problems often go untreated. That's because, he said, today there is a greater stigma associated with substance abuse than with mental illness.

A new study of mental health and substance abuse treatment expenditures released by the Substance Abuse and Mental Health Services Administration seems to bear this out.

Although it covered a period prior to implementation of the federal parity law, the study found that spending on substance abuse treatment grew more slowly than did spending for other types of mental health care between 1987 and 1997.

Adjusted for inflation, private-sector spending on substance abuse declined 0.2% during the 10-year period. In that same time, spending on other mental health care services grew 3.6%, though that figure also lagged behind the growth of private spending on overall health care, which increased at an inflation-adjusted rate of 4.1%. Furthermore, the study showed that only 36% of substance abuse treatment costs were covered privately, that is, by insurers, philanthropy or out of the pockets of patients or their families.

The study also questioned why independent specialists in mental health care and substance abuse treatment, such as psychiatrists, psychologists, counselors and social workers, receive a lower proportion of substance abuse dollars than do general physicians.

"Are these MH/SA specialists less likely to accept addiction clients than mental health clients?" the study asked. "Or are their services less likely to be covered by third-party payments?"

"Bingo!" said Joy Riley, a consultant at Watson Wyatt Worldwide in Atlanta.

"Definitely, the state of the art is more outpatient-oriented," she said, yet "most employers significantly limit the benefit to inpatient treatment."

Outpatient treatment benefits for chemical dependency usually are subject to the same limits as for other mental health care services, with sizable co-payments or limits on the number of visits, Ms. Riley said.

While most chemical dependency treatment programs start with intensive inpatient therapy, that usually lasts just three to five days. Then a patient is usually referred to an intensive outpatient therapy program that meets two to three hours a day, three or four days a week, for two weeks or more, said Joe Vollmer, supervisor of Employee & Family Counseling Services, an internal employee assistance program at Golden, Colo.-based Coors Brewing Co.

"Then there's aftercare," where the number of outpatient therapy visits gradually declines to, perhaps, one visit per week or once every two weeks, he explained.

Substance abusers "don't live in a hospital," Mr. Vollmer said. "They have to learn to deal with the triggers and the problems in the environment that they live in."

Most of Coors' insurers have adopted this philosophy, he said. Coors offers its 5,800 employees a choice from among CIGNA, Kaiser Permanente and PacifiCare HMOs and PPOs and a self-insured point-of-service plan.

Outpatient treatment also is more cost-effective, said Dr. Jerry Vaccaro, vp and corporate medical director at PacifiCare Behavioral Health in Van Nuys, Calif.

"If you take the same amount of money and spread it out over time, it's a much wiser use of resources," he said.

# Principles of Drug Addiction Treatment

More than two decades of scientific research has yielded a set of 13 fundamental principles that characterize effective drug abuse treatment. These principles are detailed in NIDA's *Principles of Drug Addiction Treatment: A Research-Based Guide.*

1. No single treatment is appropriate for all individuals. Matching treatment settings, interventions, and services to each patient's problems and needs is critical.

2. Treatment needs to be readily available. Treatment applicants can be lost if treatment is not immediately available or readily accessible.

3. Effective treatment attends to multiple needs of the individual, not just his or her drug use. Treatment must address the individual's drug use and associated medical, psychological, social, vocational, and legal problems.

4. At different times during treatment, a patient may develop a need for medical services, family therapy, vocational rehabilitation, and social and legal services.

5. Remaining in treatment for an adequate period of time is critical for treatment effectiveness. The time depends on an individual's needs. For most patients, the threshold of significant improvement is reached at about 3 months in treatment. Additional treatment can produce further progress. Programs should include strategies to prevent patients from leaving treatment prematurely.

6. Individual and/or group counseling and other behavioral therapies are critical components of effective treatment for addiction. In therapy, patients address motivation, build skills to resist drug use, replace drug-using activities with constructive and rewarding nondrug-using activities, and improve problem-solving abilities. Behavioral therapy also facilitates interpersonal relationships.

7. Medications are an important element of treatment for many patients, especially when combined with counseling and other behavioral therapies. Methadone and levo-alpha-acetylmethodol (LAAM) help persons addicted to opiates stabilize their lives and reduce their drug use. Naltrexone is effective for some opiate addicts and some patients with co-occurring alcohol dependence. Nicotine patches or gum, or an oral medication, such as buproprion, can help persons addicted to nicotine.

8. Addicted or drug-abusing individuals with coexisting mental disorders should have both disorders treated in an integrated way.

9. Medical detoxification is only the first stage of addiction treatment and by itself does little to change long-term drug use. Medical detoxification manages the acute physical symptoms of withdrawal. For some individuals it is a precursor to effective drug addiction treatment.

10. Treatment does not need to be voluntary to be effective. Sanctions or enticements in the family, employment setting, or criminal justice system can significantly increase treatment entry, retention, and success.

11. Possible drug use during treatment must be monitored continuously. Monitoring a patient's drug and alcohol use during treatment, such as through urinalysis, can help the patient withstand urges to use drugs. Such monitoring also can provide early evidence of drug use so that treatment can be adjusted.

12. Treatment programs should provide assessment for HIV/AIDS, hepatitis B and C, tuberculosis and other infectious diseases, and counseling to help patients modify or change behaviors that place them or others at risk of infection. Counseling can help patients avoid high-risk behavior and help people who are already infected manage their illness.

13. Recovery from drug addiction can be a long-term process and frequently requires multiple episodes of treatment. As with other chronic illnesses, relapses to drug use can occur during or after successful treatment episodes. Participation in self-help support programs during and following treatment often helps maintain abstinence.

Source: National Institute on Drug Abuse, *www.nida.nih.gov / DrugsofAbuse.html*

# Depressed? What Makes You Ask?[7]

BY SUZ REDFEARN
*WASHINGTON POST*, MAY 28, 2002

Last week, a top independent advisory panel recommended that primary care doctors start screening patients for depression during routine visits. Why? Because, according to the U.S. Preventive Services Task Force, providers such as family doctors and nurse practitioners currently miss and mistreat more than half of all cases of depression. In fact, of the estimated 19 million American adults who suffer from depression, as many as two-thirds aren't being treated. If primary care providers get involved, as many as 90 percent of those afflicted can get treatment, the recommendation asserts.

All of which raises questions, of course.

So next time I go to the doctor, she's going to screen me for depression?

If she's decided to follow the task force's new recommendations—which she is not compelled to do—yes.

If she's on board, she'll do one of two things during your visit: 1) Ask you whether you have felt down, depressed or hopeless over the last two weeks, and if you have felt little interest or pleasure in doing things during that time; or 2) Use a questionnaire to ask you a series of similar questions.

But don't expect universal compliance, suggests Douglas Jacobs, a Boston-area psychiatrist speaking on behalf of the American Psychiatric Association (APA). "In an ideal world, everyone would be screened by their doctor, but that's just not going to happen," he said. "Physicians are too busy."

What happens if I answer yes to the questions, or my answers to the questionnaire deem me "depressed"?

If your doctor is following the guidelines, she'll follow up with further diagnostic procedures. Most often this will consist of an interview drawing on questions designed to identify depression as defined in the *Diagnostic and Statistical Manual of Mental Disorders—Fourth Edition* (DSM-IV). Published by the APA, this is the main reference used by those in the mental health field to make diagnoses.

If your doctor makes a diagnosis of depression after that, she may prescribe antidepressant medication or refer you to a psychologist or psychiatrist.

---

## Public Awareness of Depression Growing

Americans are growing more aware of depression and its treatment, according to a recent survey from the National Mental Health Association.

The survey, released in July, found that public opinion of depression shifted in the past 10 years, with 55 percent of the general population now acknowledging that depression is a disease and not a state of mind, in comparison to 38 percent in 1991. However, nearly one-third of the participants still believed depression is a state of mind.

"Erroneous beliefs about depression fuel stigma, bad public policies and poor personal choices by those living with the illness and may impede their recovery," said Michael M. Faenza, president and chief executive officer of the mental health association.

Survey participants said depression would be best treated through therapy, exercise and a healthy diet rather than medication. In contrast, most doctors said the most effective treatment against repeated episodes of depression was long-term use of medication combined with psychotherapy and a healthy lifestyle.

About one-half of depression patients experience a relapse with the disease at some point, according to the association. However, 35 percent of the general public believed that depression can be completely cured with treatment.

"Facing up to this illness and taking personal responsibility for its treatment are vital," Faenza said. "Yet some may not acknowledge and seek treatment for depression because of negative public attitudes and misperceptions."

*Source:* Article from *The Nation's Health* September 2001. Copyright © American Public Health Association. Reproduced with permission.

Does this mean that if I think I'm depressed, I should go to my primary care doctor?

The task force says yes. According to Alfred O. Berg, a Seattle-based family physician who chairs the body that made the recommendations, most depression and anxiety disorders are now treated effectively by primary care clinicians. And most doctors are plugged into a referral network, so if your doctor feels a psychologist or a psychiatrist would better treat your condition, she can refer you to one.

Will a diagnosis of depression go on my permanent medical record?

It depends on how your doctor keeps records. Some primary care doctors don't keep records on their patients' mental health; others do. If this issue concerns you, discuss disclosure procedures with your doctor, advises Berg. "Most do go to great lengths to protect patient confidentiality," he said.

Don't insurers discriminate against people who have a history of depression?

Yes, insurers often consider depression history in their decisions. Some disability insurance carriers, life insurance companies and long-term care insurers ask for psychiatric records during the application process, and they may deny coverage if they see something they don't like. Many health insurers require people with a preexisting condition, such as depression, to wait for a specified time before they're covered for that condition; alternatively, they may exclude the condition from any coverage.

But the stigma that treatment for mental disorders once carried, even within the system, is less prevalent, says Carol Kleinman, a psychiatrist in private practice in Chevy Chase [MD]. "I do think this has improved a bit since so many people take antidepressants now, and there's a higher level of sophistication out there about depression."

How dependable are these depression tests, anyhow?

They are highly sensitive instruments, meaning they generate more false positives than false negatives. That means that in preliminary screens for depression, you may test positive if you are not depressed, but if you are depressed you are unlikely to test negative. That's so everyone who may be depressed will go to the next level and get more extensive questioning through their doctor.

> *The stigma that treatment for mental disorders once carried, even within the system, is less prevalent.*

The DSM-IV criteria for depression, on the other hand, are the gold standard for diagnosis, said Berg. That definition is somewhat mechanical, requiring a certain number of symptoms in a set of categories before a person is pronounced depressed. Screening inquiries deal with such details as the extent to which a person is feeling lonely, crying easily, applying self-blame and feeling hopeless about the future. Other parts of the test focus on physical manifestations of depression such as headaches, lower back pain and disturbances in sleeping, eating or sexual interest.

Depression screens may also help identify other conditions, such as anxiety disorders, panic attacks and substance abuse.

If I'm diagnosed with depression, will my insurer cover treatment?

Many but not all insurers will cover depression treatment delivered in a primary care setting, said Berg. Plans that offer coverage for prescription drugs usually cover medications for depression, but some drugs may carry higher co-pays than others. If you are referred to a psychologist or psychiatrist, your plan may offer strict limitations on whom you may see and how much and what kind of treatment will be covered. Call your insurance company for details.

Are there any online tests I can use to check myself out?

Doctors generally don't consider this a good idea. Their thinking is that you could disregard the test if you don't like the results rather than getting the treatment you might need. Also, docs feel that people who are depressed often aren't thinking clearly, which could make self-assessment troublesome. That said, the Zung Self-Assessment Depression Scale, which the task force recommended that doctors use in initial depression screening, is available for consumers by going to www.prozac.com/SelfAssessmentTest.jsp. This is a commercial site hosted by Eli Lilly, the maker of Prozac. Click on "Zung Scale Self-Assessment Test" and then on "click here just to take the test," which permits you to take the test anonymously.

Didn't *The Post* just run a big story that said placebos are just as effective as antidepressant medications in treating depression? What's up with that?

Recent analyses have shown that in clinical tests, some patients getting sugar pills reported better outcomes than patients getting the real antidepressants. And one researcher has documented that people reporting benefits from a placebo had measurable changes in brain activity of the sort often associated with improvements from depression. This appears related to the fact that in most studies, subjects getting the placebo were getting care and attention from health professionals as part of the process. The result is controversial. In its review of literature, the task force concluded that antidepressants are "clearly" more effective than placebos for depression.

I don't like taking drugs. Doesn't therapy relieve depression, too?

Recent studies conducted at the University of Pennsylvania and Vanderbilt University have shown that a form of treatment called cognitive therapy—in which a patient is helped to understand, recognize and reduce the effect of his or her irrational thoughts and behaviors—is at least as effective as medication for long-term treatment of severe depression. The task force concludes that therapy appears to be effective, but often takes longer than treatment with medication. Other studies have shown that therapy and drugs together work better for many patients than either one alone, but the task force did not find this research conclusive.

The topic is also controversial. Geoffrey M. Reed, assistant executive director for professional development at the American Psychological Association, which represents psychologists, said that patients tend to prefer psychotherapy, but managed care companies prefer that doctors treat the depressed with medicine. Berg adds that in his experience, many times drugs work more quickly.

# II.  The Business of Health Care

# Editor's Introduction

I n recent years, the business of health care has received at least as much attention as the quality and availability of health care. Politicians, employers, and medical professionals seem more concerned with how to pay for treatment once people become ill than with how to maintain good health and prevent illness. Most will agree that paying for quality health care is one of the greatest challenges facing Americans today, and this topic is the subject of the book's second chapter. Millions of Americans are without health insurance (most of them women, the elderly, and the poor), and the number continues to rise. For years, Congress, the White House, advocacy groups, and state legislatures have been trying to devise a solution to the health insurance problem, but to no avail. Congress's reluctance to support a plan for universal health insurance in 1994 demonstrates what a contentious issue this has become. With the rising costs of medications, increasing premiums from health maintenance organizations (HMOs), the inability of many employers to provide adequate insurance, and the constant threats to Medicare and Medicaid, there seems to be no way out of the black hole.

The first article, "What Price Health Care Quality?" by Len M. Nichols, examines the problems facing Medicare and Medicaid, and how quality is often sacrificed to cost. Without universal health insurance, Americans must find other means to pay for quality coverage. For the uninsured and many senior citizens, that method is through government-subsidized Medicare and Medicaid. Nichols discusses the differences between the care offered through these government programs and private and employer-sponsored health insurance plans. An accompanying sidebar defines both Medicare and Medicaid and those who qualify for each.

One reason the number of uninsured is growing is because of the economic downturn of the last two years. "New Partnership Campaigns for 'Covering the Uninsured'" announces the formation of the Covering the Uninsured coalition to help those experiencing financial difficulties pay for health care. This coalition is comprised of different advocacy groups, including the AARP, the AFL-CIO, and the American Medical Association. As they work to solve the problem of uninsurance in the United States, they also strive to increase awareness about this pressing issue.

While Americans wait for the federal government to devise a program for universal health insurance, several states are conceiving their own plans to help their citizens afford quality health care. A new type of health plan that is being tested in California is a tiered plan that gives members the opportunity to save money by choosing their provider's "A list" hospitals or paying more by going with a "B" or "C list" facility. Laura B. Benko considers this new plan in her article "HMOs Aren't Shedding Tiers." Under this system, employers, as well as employees, are expected to reap the benefits of quality care with cheaper health insurance.

PPOs (preferred-provider organizations) are becoming the new wave in health insurance and now boast more members than HMOs. Unlike HMOs, PPOs allow their members to use in- and out-of-network providers, thereby giving patients more of a selection. Lori Chordas, in "Step Right Up," looks at this new phenomenon, compares PPOs to HMOs, and discusses why more people are making the switch to PPOs.

Another alternative to an HMO is a Medical Savings Account (MSA). MSAs benefit small businesses and those who are self-employed by enabling them to buy large deductible major medical policies for half of what they would pay to an HMO. Steve Pielacha discusses the difference between MSAs and HMOs in "Medical Savings Account: The Health Insurance Secret." According to Pielacha, MSAs would provide Americans with precisely what polls show they want—"control and choices when it comes to their health."

One of the most important issues in health insurance deals with insuring critically ill patients. Many employer-sponsored insurance providers do not cover critical illnesses, or if they do, coverage is limited. Rudy M. Yandrick, in "Bridge over Troubled Waters," discusses a new type of insurance—CII, or critical illness insurance—geared towards critically ill patients and their families. He talks about the benefits and what to look for when considering this type of insurance.

The final article in this chapter, "The Bill for Rights," discusses the implications of the currently debated Patients' Bill of Rights, which, among other things, would include giving patients the opportunity to sue their health providers. With a large number of people supporting such a bill, Carl E. Schneider offers seven reasons to be skeptical of it.

# What Price Health Care Quality?[1]

By Len M. Nichols
*USA Today Magazine*, January 1999

As Medicaid and Medicare adopt the cost-control techniques used by the private sector, including managed care and competitive billing, the uninsured will find it even more difficult to afford medical treatment. [See "Important Health Care Terms" at the end of this book for explanations of Medicare and Medicaid.]

After Congress rejected universal health insurance coverage in 1994, much of the nation's health policy attention turned to quality assurance. The hundreds of specific clinical requirements for health plans introduced by state legislatures and Congress reflect widespread concern that too much access and service quality are being sacrificed for cost containment in the private sector. At the same time, some policymakers are demanding that the largest public programs, Medicare and Medicaid, emulate private-sector cost savings, the very ones that have sparked the current concern over quality. Therefore, two key health policy challenges for the future will be maintaining a high level of quality as costs are contained in public programs and striking the right policy balance in monitoring and regulating the quality of health care in the private sector.

After 10 years of double-digit health insurance premium inflation in the 1980s, the current decade has seen a steady decline in the rate of private premium growth. For example, premiums for employer-sponsored insurance increased by about 0.5% and total national health spending rose at 4.4% in 1996, the smallest rate of growth since 1960. Slower national health care cost growth means that more resources are available for other deskable uses. These cost containment successes widely are attributed to the spread of managed care.

Yet, some consumers and policymakers have come to fear the techniques that managed care health plans use to contain costs, such as limiting access to specific providers and services and creating incentives for providers to curtail access to care. These techniques can cut costs, but risk reducing actual or perceived quality of care. The legislative proposals and the recent presidential commission on quality in health care are responses to this perceived risk.

---

1. Article by Len M. Nichols from *USA Today* January 1999. Copyright © Society for the Advancement of Education. Reprinted with permission.

Governments directly purchase health care for almost 27% of Americans through Medicare (a Federal program for the elderly and disabled) and Medicaid (a joint Federal-state program for the poor). On behalf of these beneficiaries, the public sector directly pays for almost 40% of all health services delivered in this country, and the public share of health care finance is even higher if tax subsidies for private employment-related insurance are counted. These coverage and cost percentages make clear that the elderly and the poor are less healthy than the rest of Americans. No one disputes that cost growth must be curtailed in these large public programs. Combined, they represent more than $350,000,000,000 of annual government spending.

During the 1980s, Medicare costs rose in real terms at more than seven percent and Medicaid expenses at about six percent a year—historical growth rates that clearly were unsustainable. Spending has slowed somewhat, but still is faster than real gross domestic product increases of 2.8%. Recent spending growth reductions in Medicare largely are due to fee-for-service payment reforms, while Medicaid's successes mostly reflect the end of enrollment expansions and the exhaustion of "Medicaid maximization" strategies, whereby many states substitute Federal for state health care dollars.

The 1997 Balanced Budget Act achieved some Medicare savings and, to a much lesser extent, reduced Medicaid spending, but the budget agreement did little to address the long-run demographic problem that threatens the adequacy of Medicare funding: the decline in the worker/beneficiary ratio from the current three-to-one to two-to-one by the time the last baby boomers are retired. As a result, many inside and outside of Congress are proposing long-term structural changes to both programs that will institutionalize cost containment incentives. Managed care and the increased health plan competition that managed care makes possible are central to these structural proposals.

The revolution in delivery patterns (less in-patient and more ambulatory care), spurred in part by 1980s Medicare payment reforms and lately by the demands of employers in the private sector, has created an excess supply of hospital beds and physicians. These developments have forced many health providers into price competition for the first time.

With declines in hospital admission rates and average lengths of stay, average hospital occupancy rates are below 63%, and recent estimates of the physician surplus suggest that the nation needs about 30% fewer doctors than are graduating each year. Price competition is inevitable in this environment, even in health care markets that successfully have resisted price competition in the past.

Provider price competition has many virtues, which managed health care plans, large self-insured employers, big and small employer coalitions, and some state governments have been quick to exploit. The provider price competition spawned by excess capacity largely is responsible for the slowdown in private-sector premiums, and the lower premiums that managed care plans can offer largely are responsible for their increasing share of the health insurance market. The downside of health care provider price competition is less obvious.

### Subsidizing the Uninsured

Traditionally, acute hospital care for the uninsured has been financed through implicit cross-subsidies. That is, hospitals would charge paying (i.e., insured) patients more than the average cost of serving them, and the surplus thus extracted was used to finance care for the uninsured. This cross-subsidy was facilitated by the preponderance of nonprofit (and public) hospitals that, by law, could not distribute any surplus they might earn to stockholders, but instead were expected to utilize any surplus in ways that benefited their communities at large.

Uncompensated hospital care has averaged about six percent of total hospital expenses each year since 1984. That figure masks the fact that a disproportionate share of uncompensated care is provided by hospitals (especially public teaching ones) that serve large percentages of Medicaid patients. Uncompensated care as a percentage of expenses approaches 20% for some major public teaching hospitals. This level of charity care requires direct subsidies or a significant markup on charges to insured patients. A more competitive market for insured patients will reduce hospitals' flexibility to charge more than true costs to any patients, private or public. This will be especially true as public programs move away from their rigid, formula-based payment methods and use competitive bidding with providers and managed care plans.

As public payors such as the Medicaid and Medicare programs adopt the cost-control devices and techniques (managed care and competitive bidding) used by the private sector, the traditional, hidden sources of financing care for the uninsured will dry up. This scenario will force a policy choice between developing new and explicit funding sources to finance uncompensated care, expanding coverage to the uninsured through new government subsidy programs, and further restricting care for the uninsured. This choice will become more salient if the number of uninsured continues to grow. Care for the uninsured has been more difficult to finance with implicit cross-subsidies than has acute hospital care.

What happens to quality with all this emphasis on costs and competitive health markets? State governments always have played a major role in setting quality standards for health care through licensing and certification requirements for health professionals, insurers, and managed care plans. As evidenced by state and Federal legislative interest in imposing mandated clinical requirements on health plans (e.g., specified lengths of hospital stays after childbirth or certain surgeries), the boundaries of allowable private-sector trade-offs between cost and quality are being redrawn.

A real danger, however, is that well-intentioned legislators may overreact to heightened concern about quality in managed care plans and dictate clinical rules that stifle managed care plans' ability to reduce costs while maintaining or even enhancing the quality of care. Fee-for-service medicine and indemnity health plans never were held to the standards currently being discussed for managed care. For instance, many health insurance purchasers have begun requiring plans to report health outcome measures and the results of patient satisfaction surveys. A few buyers even provide this information to consumers so they can make informed choices about which plan to select. The general policy goal is to make quality-cost trade-offs clear, not to force "one quality fits all" medicine, for that one quality level may be either more than some people can afford or less than what others are willing to pay for.

The success of competitive market approaches to health policy ultimately rests on informed consumer choice. Consumers' use and understanding of quality measures may differ, though, from those of

---

### *The success of competitive market approaches to health policy ultimately rests on informed consumer choice.*

---

employers who select most plans for their employees and from those of health professionals who actually know what these measures do and don't mean. How consumers utilize quality measures surely will evolve as their use and dissemination by health plans and organized purchasers change over time.

A focus on quality and quality reporting is positive, but the pressure on managed care plans to "do well" on measurable outcomes may skew provider resources away from those dimensions of quality that are harder to measure, but may be equally or more important to the average plan enrollee (e.g., discomfort during recovery).

This "quality information" dimension of competitive health plan markets still is in its infancy. Consumers, legislators, employers, and public-sector program managers need to remember this before demanding too much too soon, or believing they have received more predictive information than actually is possible to produce at the present time.

Another problem with relying too heavily on quality measures is that public health program beneficiaries such as the elderly and the low-income population may have criteria for quality care that differ from those of the employed non-elderly population, and thus may process and use available information in different ways. For example, the elderly may care more about comfort and may not want to sort through complicated comparison reports.

Although Medicare and Medicaid may benefit from the recent lessons learned in private health care markets, there are three reasons they can not behave exactly like private employers or employer coalitions do when purchasing health insurance. First, public programs must serve all eligible beneficiaries, not just some. Medicare and Medicaid can not segment themselves away from the sickest beneficiaries, as private insurance plans and employers often do. Thus, government programs do not have the same paths to cost reduction used by the private sector, some of which involve merely shifting costs to government.

Second, public payors must be mindful of the effects that aggressive purchasing power can have. Urban public teaching hospitals provide vital services for economically disadvantaged populations. As competition forces these hospitals to reduce prices for paying patients, it drains their traditional financing streams. When this happens, other public funding for these services must be found or the consequences of care rationing will become increasingly apparent, both in suburban emergency rooms and in the local media.

Finally, public program beneficiaries may need a more active ombudsman as their purchasing agent than do the employed non-elderly who are making choices among managed care plans in an employer-sponsored setting. The principles of informed competition continue to apply to public health care programs, but policy-makers who set the rules of that competition for public dollars should keep in mind the specific needs of these beneficiaries.

# New Partnership Campaigns for "Covering the Uninsured"[2]

*NATION'S HEALTH*, APRIL 2002

Thirteen diverse national organizations joined together in February to seek solutions for the high number of uninsured families in the United States.

The organizations formed the Covering the Uninsured coalition, which includes the Robert Wood Johnson Foundation, AARP, U.S. Chamber of Commerce, AFL-CIO, American Medical Association, Families USA and American Nurses Association.

"There are too many families who suffer because our nation has ignored the crisis of the uninsured, leaving them to deal on their own with the costs and consequences of this crisis when sickness or injury hits their home," said AFL-CIO President John J. Sweeney at a February news conference in Washington, D.C. "We are here today to pledge our organizations to covering the uninsured. Our nation's leaders should do the same."

The coalition unveiled a $10 million public education campaign that includes print and Internet advertising, two television ads and a new Web site, <*www.coveringtheuninsured.org*>.

The campaign "will give voice to this quiet crisis," said Steven A. Schroeder, MD, president and chief executive officer of the Robert Wood Johnson Foundation.

In 2000, 39 million Americans were uninsured, and that number appeared to increase in 2001, as economic troubles led to numerous job layoffs.

About 2 million Americans lost their health insurance in 2001, the largest one-year increase in almost a decade, according to new data released in February by Families USA.

About half of the increase occurred from September through December, reflecting the impact of Sept. 11, said Ron Pollack, executive director of Families USA.

Pollack added that the numbers are conservative because they do not include the effect of increased health costs and cutbacks in state Medicaid programs.

A survey conducted for Covering the Uninsured showed that many more Americans were afraid of losing their coverage: 43 percent of those surveyed in January said they believed that their or their spouse's employer might cut back or eliminate some health care benefits within the next year.

2. Article from *The Nation's Health* April 2002. Copyright © American Public Health Association. Reprinted with permission.

For the first time since the early 1990s, there was a double-digit measurement of concern about unemployment: Eleven percent of survey participants said they were concerned about unemployment and the lack of jobs.

"This is a health crisis of massive proportions, and it's getting worse," Schroeder said. "We know that the uninsured will live sicker and die younger."

Representatives from the organizations did not go into specifics on how to solve the uninsurance problem, admitting that they don't all share the same opinions on a solution. However, they said they are willing to work together to draw attention to the crisis and seek solutions. The representatives signed a proclamation that outlines the uninsurance problem and declares that "we have come together from diverse perspectives to seek solutions to one of America's greatest problems."

"They are rising above (their policy differences) to achieve a greater goal," Schroeder said. "And we encourage the American people and their representatives to join us as we come together to meet our challenges and solve this problem."

APHA supports a comprehensive, universal health care system under 2000 policy.

# HMOs Aren't Shedding Tiers[3]

By Laura B. Benko
*Modern Healthcare*, December 3, 2001

After readily embracing tiered drug formularies as a way to contain costs, health plans now are applying the same concept to providers.

At least three large California HMOs are exploring a new type of health plan that promises big savings—but only if patients go to a discount "A list" of hospitals within the plan's regular provider network. Those who choose to go to a "B list" provider will be forced to pay several times more.

All three plans are promoting this tiered model as a way to cut employers' expenses by forcing workers to be more cost-conscious when deciding where to get hospital care. But in addition to stemming hospital costs, such efforts ultimately could give insurers renewed leverage when negotiating contracts with providers, many of which have been enjoying increased clout at the bargaining table.

Santa Ana-based PacifiCare Health Systems is rolling out a new product called the Select Hospital Plan to medium and large employers in California, where it has some 1.7 million enrollees. Health Net and Blue Cross of California, both based in Woodland Hills, are working quietly on similar products. Neither one, however, has set a launch date.

Under the Select Hospital Plan, which will be available Jan. 1, members who choose to receive care from PacifiCare's list of "select" hospitals—facilities that have agreed to provide services at cheaper rates—won't pay any out-of-pocket fees. But those who opt to go to the other hospitals in PacifiCare's network will be socked with copayments of $100, $250 or $400 per visit, depending on the cost-sharing arrangement employers choose.

## Passing Along Costs

Premium savings for employers are expected to range from 5% to 20%, says PacifiCare spokeswoman Cheryl Randolph. The insurer predicts 10% of its customers will transfer to the lower-cost plan next year.

---

Facing double-digit rate increases, "employers are looking for ways to pass more of their benefit costs down to employees, who basically have been shielded by $5 and $10 copays," Randolph said. "What we are trying to do is tie the members' medical costs to the true cost of care."

The tiered HMO is reminiscent of a PPO in that members are encouraged to choose from a network of "preferred" providers. But unlike PPOs, the tiered plan ranks providers within its own network.

*"If hospitals don't cut a deal, they face the possibility of losing business."*—Glenn Smith, Watson Wyatt Worldwide

About a third of the 300 hospitals that PacifiCare contracts with statewide have agreed to join the program. The list is dominated by California's largest hospital chains: Tenet Healthcare Corp., Sutter Health System, Catholic Healthcare West, HCA, Sharp HealthCare and Scripps Health.

Absent from the list, though, are some large standalone hospitals, including 849-bed Cedars-Sinai Medical Center in Los Angeles and the 528-bed University of California-Davis Medical Center in Sacramento. The latter is still in talks with PacifiCare.

"There are a number of factors to consider," says UC-Davis spokeswoman Bonnie Hyatt. "For one thing, is it financially feasible for us (to join)? And if we don't join, how many patients would be affected?"

It's through this sort of dilemma that tiered health plans could provide PacifiCare and other insurers with a new bargaining chip at contract time. The plans give HMOs the power to steer potentially large numbers of patients toward hospitals that are willing to offer them discounts—and away from those that balk.

"If hospitals don't cut a deal, they face the possibility of losing business," says Glenn Smith, a healthcare consultant with Watson Wyatt Worldwide in San Francisco. "Basically, what these health plans are saying is, 'We've steered business toward you, but if you don't deliver, we'll relegate you to the B list.'"

## Targeting Hospital Spending

In addressing hospital costs, health plans are trying to rein in one of the leading causes of medical inflation.

According to a report released in September by the Center for Studying Health System Change, healthcare spending rose 7.2% in 2000—the largest jump in a decade—with hospital spending accounting for nearly half, or 43%, of the total increase.

While inpatient hospital spending rose just 2.8% last year, the increase was up from a 1.6% jump in 1999. This rise reverses a trend from 1994 to 1998 when inpatient spending actually dropped by as much as 5.3% a year.

# Top 25 HMOs ranked by Medicare enrollment

As of July 1, 2000

| | | Medicare enrollment | Total HMO enrollment | Primary-care physicians | Specialty-care physicians | Year founded | Type of firm |
|---|---|---|---|---|---|---|---|
| 1 | PacifiCare of California<br>Cypress, Calif. (714) 952-1121 | 566,588 | 2,390,277 | 11,117 | 19,020 | 1978 | For profit |
| 2 | Kaiser Foundation Health Plan Inc.,<br>No. CA region Oakland, Calif. (510) 987-1000 | 320,548 | 3,023,925 | 2,464 | 3,504 | 1946 | Not for profit |
| 3 | Humana Medical Plan Inc.<br>Miramar, Fla. (305) 626-5616 | 281,823 | 621,051 | 8,688 | NA | 1973 | For profit |
| 4 | Kaiser Foundation Health Plan Inc.,<br>So. CA region Pasadena, Calif. (626) 405-5000 | 279,654 | 2,972,898 | 1,947 | 2,078 | 1943 | Not for profit |
| 5 | Keystone Health Plan West<br>Pittsburgh, Pa. (412) 544-7000 | 151,822 | 451,869 | 2,621 | 4,731 | 1987 | For profit |
| 6 | Health Options Inc.<br>Jacksonville, Fla. (904) 905-3111 | 151,628 | 924,854 | 4,632 | 12,716 | 1980 | For profit |
| 7 | United States Health Care Systems of PA<br>Blue Bell, Pa. (800) 872-3862 | 132,124 | 790,366 | 6,719 | 13,712 | 1976 | For profit |
| 8 | Humana Health Plan Inc.<br>Louisville, Ky. (502) 580-5001 | 129,988 | 787,930 | 710 | 1,430 | 1987 | For profit |
| 9 | Keystone Health Plan East Inc.<br>Philadelphia, Pa. (215) 241-2400 | 127,504 | 1,078,591 | 8,149 | 15,060 | 1987 | For profit |
| 10 | Health Net of California<br>Woodland Hills, Calif. (818) 676-7214 | 122,224 | 2,210,252 | 11,924 | 25,745 | 1979 | For profit |
| 11 | Tufts Health Plan<br>Waltham, Mass. (781) 466-9400 | 104,300 | 637,029 | 6,050 | 11,211 | 1982 | Not for profit |
| 12 | HIP Health Plan of New York<br>New York, N.Y. (212) 630-5000 | 102,805 | 770,417 | 5,447 | 7,972 | 1947 | Not for profit |
| 13 | PacifiCare of Arizona Inc.<br>Phoenix, Ariz. (602) 244-2707 | 98,448 | 201,093 | 1,180 | 2,274 | 1986 | For profit |
| 14 | Aetna U.S. Healthcare Inc.<br>Fairfield, N.J. (800) 872-3862 | 89,835 | 883,175 | 5,303 | 8,703 | 1983 | For profit |
| 15 | Blue Shield of California Access+HMO<br>San Francisco, Calif. (415) 229-5000 | 80,243 | 985,159 | 10,122 | 17,763 | 1988 | Not for profit |
| 16 | Oxford Health Plans of New York<br>New York, N.Y. (800) 889-7622 | 77,514 | 1,033,183 | 9,527 | 21,873 | 1986 | For profit |
| 17 | U.S. Healthcare Inc.<br>Uniondale, N.Y. (516) 794-6565 | 71,670 | 907,465 | 7,500 | 15,530 | 1986 | For profit |
| 18 | PacifiCare of Colorado Inc.<br>Englewood, Colo. (800) 877-6685 | 67,383 | 380,985 | 1,424 | 2,957 | 1988 | For profit |
| 19 | PacifiCare of Texas<br>Dallas, Texas (972) 206-1693 | 67,288 | 195,463 | 2,730 | 5,431 | 1986 | For profit |
| 20 | Regence HMO Oregon/Health Maintenance<br>of Oregon Inc. Portland, Ore. (503) 225-5221 | 64,914 | 277,488 | 2,291 | 5,755 | 1977 | Not for profit |
| 21 | Aetna U.S. Healthcare of California Inc.<br>San Ramon, Calif. (925) 543-9000 | 63,105 | 707,533 | 12,218 | 24,057 | 1978 | For profit |
| 22 | Anthem BCBS-Anthem HMO<br>Mason, Ohio (513) 336-4077 | 62,893 | 238,769 | 5,709 | 6,133 | 1974 | For profit |
| 23 | Intergroup of Arizona Inc.<br>Tucson, Ariz. (800) 289-2818 | 59,356 | 349,024 | 1,380 | 2,760 | 1981 | For profit |
| 24 | Group Health Cooperative<br>Spokane, Wash. (509) 241-7423 | 59,170 | 575,629 | 1,015 | 4,914 | 1946 | Not for profit |
| 25 | United HealthCare of the Midwest Inc.<br>Maryland Heights, Mo. (314) 592-7000 | 58,307 | 528,874 | 2,193 | 4,475 | 1986 | For profit |

NA=not available

MHE Source: The InterStudy Competitive Edge (Minneapolis), 2001.

*Source:* Table by Jean Appleby from *Managed Healthcare Executive* January 2002. Copyright © *Managed Healthcare Executive.* Reprinted with permission.

Indeed, these new products represent an about-face from HMOs' recent push to lure customers by providing fewer restrictions, more services and broader networks. That strategy, health plans say, has led to higher costs—and higher premiums—because enrollees have lacked any financial incentive to choose lower-cost care options.

"If HMOs are going to hold the line on costs, they need to recognize that they can't make every provider available to their members at the same cost," says Health Net spokesman Brad Kieffer, who declined to comment on the company's new health plan other than to say that it would be introduced "as soon as possible."

Health plans are banking on the belief that patients will be willing to travel a bit farther to get a better deal. State law requires HMOs to offer providers within 15 miles or a 30-minute drive, but members can elect to drive farther, says Blue Cross spokesman Michael Chee.

"It's based entirely on member choice," Chee says. "As a member, I can decide to go to hospital A, which may be a little closer, or to hospital B, which gives me a price break."

Consumer advocates, however, are taking a more cautious attitude toward tiered HMOs.

Members in PacifiCare's new health plan will have to choose a physician who uses a "select" hospital, and many people may not be willing to switch doctors, says Beth Cappell, an advocate for Oakland-based consumer group Health Access California.

"The jury is still out on how successful these types of plans will be," Cappell says.

To be sure, the network-within-a-network concept isn't unique to the Golden State. Tufts Health Plan of Waltham, Mass., plans to begin offering a similar type of product, called the Choice Co-Pay Plan, to Massachusetts employees next year. Under the plan, the inpatient admission charge paid by enrollees will be twice as much if they receive care at an academic medical center instead of at a community hospital.

But the idea seems to be catching on with particular speed in California, where insurers have been increasingly stymied at the bargaining table by big hospital systems.

Blue Cross, for instance, was forced to make significant concessions to Sutter Health System this year after a lengthy skirmish over reimbursement rates. Analysts said the 2 million-member insurer would have lost much of its clout in Northern California had it failed to renew its contract with Sacramento-based Sutter, which operates 26 of the region's hospitals.

Whether Sutter will choose to become a part of Blue Cross' upcoming "A list" remains to be seen. But Bill Gleeson, a spokesman for the hospital system, says Sutter will opt out of any health plan that doesn't offer adequate reimbursements, regardless of how many patients it may lose.

"The days of contracting with as many health plans as possible are over," Gleeson says. "Healthcare organizations are having to make increasingly difficult decisions. It's become a matter of survival."

# Step Right Up[4]

By Lori Chordas
*Best's Review*, March 2002

CareFirst Blue Cross Blue Shield knows how to pick a winner. The company, which serves customers in Maryland, Delaware. northern Virginia and Washington, D.C., was the first carrier in its region to offer a preferred-provider organization. Since 1996, its PPO membership has doubled, increasing by more than 600,000 individuals.

Health maintenance organizations, the enrollment darlings of the 1980s and early- to mid-'90s, are losing members in what is being called the "decade of the PPO." Unlike HMOs, which require that individuals see a primary-care physician, remain in network for coverage and obtain referrals prior to seeing specialists. PPOs allow members to see providers both within and outside a network.

Today, an estimated 100 million people in the United States belong to PPOs, which enroll far more members than do HMOs and are growing at a more rapid rate, according to the National Committee for Quality Assurance, a nonprofit organization that evaluates and reports on the quality of managed-care organizations.

The cost gap that once drove some employers to forgo PPOs for less expensive HMO products is now narrowing, and many insurers are confident that the trend of PPO enrollment growth will continue. HMOs remain in the fray, however, and to compete, they are adopting many features found in PPO-style plans.

## On the Rise

PPO enrollment has increased to 48% of all workers' health insurance from 35% just three years ago, according to a survey commissioned by the Henry J. Kaiser Family Foundation, a nonprofit organization focused on major healthcare issues. HMO membership declined to 23% from 27% during the same period.

Location and company size are key factors in enrollment patterns of the health-care models. While HMOs continue to dominate the western United States with 42% of the market compared with 29% nationally. PPOs have a greater market share, in northeastern and mid-Atlantic states. HMOs have the largest market share (37%)

among business with more than 5,000 employees, while PPOs have nearly one-half the market share in all firm sizes except the smallest and largest companies.

> *"People like PPOs because managed care hasn't worked."*—Barry Scheur, The Oath Inc.

Humana is another commercial carries that has seen a steady rise in PPO enrollment over the past several years. As of November, Hamana had more than 1.2 million members enrolled in some type of PPO product." I think a PPO is a good fit for many, consumers, because it allows them to access the provider of their choice and take advantage of arrangements we have with them," said Beth Bierbower, vice president of product development for the Louisville, KY-based organization.

**Reasons for Growth**

More choices, freedom from having to obtain services within a network, and greater flexibility are the main reasons nonrestrictive PPOs have become the clear-cut leaders among health-care models today,

Unfulfilled promises made by HMOs to offer more choices and better standards of care also have contributed to the rise in PPOs enrollment. "HMOs started with a lot of promise in the mid-to late '70s that preventative care and a range of prevention techniques would allow providers to take better care of patients," said Jim Jacobson, a partner with Holland and Knight's National Health Law Group in Boston. But HMOs haven't fulfilled that promise because the focus shifted in the 1980s from preventative care to cost-containment methods he said.

The consumer backlash against managed care and negative publicity surrounding HMOs have been linked to the model's decline. People find the word "managed" and the concept of health care being controlled unfavorable, said Barbara Benevento, senior vice president for health business for Blue Cross Blue Shield of Florida.

"People like PPOs because managed care hasn't worked," said Barry Scheur, chairman of Boston-based The Oath Inc., a private equity corporation that acquires distressed and undervalued provider-owned HMOs. "It doesn't mean it can't work; it just doesn't work."

"Primary-care physicians participating in managed-care plans often operate like mills, rushing patients through visits with barely enough time for the patient to ask questions," Jacobson said. This is because manage-care reimbursements (capitation, withholds, bonuses/penalities) typically provide a financial incentive to primary-care physicians, and even many specialists, to restrict or withhold care coordination, follow-up care, referrals to other providers and even the physician's own time with the patient, he said. "The more patients the PCP sees under managed care, the more money he or she makes, but unfortunately, the poorer quality care the patient receives." The key to turning around this perverse incentive is to transpose cost-containment incentives into quality incentives, but only a few HMOs have taken that leap of faith, he added. PPOs. on the other hand, do not usually capitate physicians or provide other incentives to withhold care.

Much of the success of PPOs was fueled by the Blue Cross Blue Shield system, particularly with the creation of its Blue Card Program, said Joseph Berardo, chief marketing officer of the preferred-provider organization MultiPlan Inc. The electronic program allows national employers, regardless of where they live or work, access to Blue Cross Blue Shield providers. "Because you have success of the Blues in most markets, other commercial and regional carriers developed a lot of products to compete with the broad network of BCBS," he said. MultiPlan has created network solutions and programs that complete directly with the BCBS Blue Card Program on a regional and national basis. These programs include a Triple Option Program, which comprises a three-tiered approach to coverage, and MultiPlan Plus, a program offering clients more enhanced product offerings in targeted geographics areas.

## Closing the Gap

The anticipated double-digit rise in health-care costs is likely to bolster the popularity of PPO plans. Increases of 13% to 16%. depending on the type of health plan, are projected to hit the industry soon, according to Hewitt Associates LLC, a global management consulting and outsourcing firm. Hewitt projects tile average health plan will cost $5,524 per employee this year, up from $4,778 in 2001. In addition, employees will pay between $186 and $463 per month for health coverage this year.

Global consulting firm Watson Wyatt predicts that health-care companies' increases will be greater than originally expected for many corporate-benefit plans this year, due to the recessionary environment and the impact of the Sept. 11 catastrophe. Watson Wyatt expects to see corporate health-care benefit costs increase by more than 15% this year.

"The days of HMOs' competitive advantage in the market through pricing is now a thing of the past," said Alan Katz, senior vice president of individual and small group sales for WellPoint in Thousand Oaks, California.

In 2000, employers reported for the first time a greater increase in the average cost of their HMO plans than in PPO models, up from 7.7% to 9.6%, according to the American Association of Preferred Provider Organizations. The gap between the costs of covering an employee through an HMO and through a PPO narrowed to about $300, and HMO plan sponsors are paying now for the deep discounts of 1996 and 1997.

According to the association, factors that have a greater impact on HMO costs and are contributing to the counterintuitive trend include:

- higher administrative overhead;
- tougher negotiating by providers on both reimbursement and compliance with administrative requirements; and
- HMO populations that are less healthy.

PPOs are actually growing in cost at a slower rate than HMOs, said Randall Abbott, a senior consultant with Watson Wyatt. For years, most PPO and point-of-service plans had annual cost increases of 6% to 8%. During the last two years, however, the rate was significantly higher, he said. In a recent survey, Watson Wyatt found that employers expected their health-care costs in 2001 to go up 13.6% with indemnity plans projected to increase about 14.4%, HMOs 13.9% and PPOs 13.7%. "This is showing that the gap in cost escalation between the two models—PPOs and HMOs—has now virtually eroded," said Abbott.

---

### *PPOs are actually growing in cost at a slower rate than HMOs.*

---

Geography is also a factor in the cost differential between the two products. In the West, HMOs offer significantly lower costs, according to the association. But there is little difference in costs between the models in midwestern states.

As the traditional underwriting cycle, which in broad terms means three years of profitable growth followed by a three-year downturn, reasserts itself, health plans are seeing the need to increase rates rapidly on all products to keep up with medical cost increases, said WellPoint's Katz, who added that the industry is currently in all upside of the cycle. HMOs, in many ways, have been the hardest hit by the cycle, because they offer rich benefits and are being weaned from capitation, he said. Also, providers are pushing more risk back onto managed-care companies. As a result, HMO rate increases are in many cases surpassing those of PPOs, Katz said.

While PPO costs remain a hit higher than those of HMOs, consumers' desire for choices takes precedence over paying higher prices. A recent Mercer/Foster Higgins study found that while HMO costs are $267.90 per employee per month on average, PPOs have been able to offer high-quality care with choices for the consumer for only $291.17 per month per employee.

### HMOs' Transformation

To complete with the open accessibility and freedom of choice offered by PPO products, HMOs are changing portions of their requirements to parallel PPO plan offerings.

In the past, HMOs tried to become more like PPOs through point-of-service plans, which allow members to go outside the HMO network. "HMOs created these plans in direct opposition to PPO growth," said Ken Linde, chief executive officer of Bethesda. Md.-based Destiny Health, a privately held insurance company. Destiny offers a health plan that allows members to keep the money in their personal medical funds if they leave the plan rather than the "use-it-or-lose-it" proposition found in traditional PPOs. While some consumers found point-of-service plans a favorable alternative to PPOs, most preferred PPO products because the plans paid more in fee schedules without nearly as many restrictions, Linde said.

"Many HMO companies are now scrambling to come up with PPO strategies and plans," said WellPoint's Katz. Over the past several years, WellPoint has shifted many of its products into hybrid plans, which combine elements of HMOs, such as preventative-care mechanisms, and PPO strategies, such as high-cost sharing and coinsurance. WellPoint customers are expressing increased interest in these plans.

In addition, many HMOs have lifted referal requirements and taken on a more "open access" approach by doing away with requirements that members must select a, primary-care physician, or gatekeeper. Humana recently changed its Humana/ChoiceCare Plan HMO by lifting referral requirements and allowing members to go directly to any specialist within the network.

Blue Shield of California, based in San Francisco, added direct access to specialists in its HMO in 1997 so members can see a specialist in a medical group or individual physician practice organization by paying a $30 copay. "Our perspective was that we should be bringing innovations to the HMO in order to meet consumers' needs," said Ken Wood, executive vice president and chief operating officer.

Some observers believe there eventually will be a blending of the two products. "Five years from now, if someone talks about HMOs and PPOs, it may be unclear as to what is being talked about, because the models will have blended enough to that those kinds of labels will be less meaningful," said WellPoint's Katz. Instead, the blended plans will feature a tradeoff between fixed costs (premiums) and variable costs (out-of-pocket costs), as well as between benefits and coverage designs that promote preventative care, often found in HMO products, and benefits in which going to a particular provider will be less costly to members, he said.

Some insurers, however, believe HMOs will not transform into more PPO-like products, but will remain one of many separate portfolio choices offered to consumers. When Blue Cross Blue Shield of Florida recently removed several restrictions, including mandatory authorization and referral requirements, from its HMO products, the result was a dramatic rise in costs, Florida Blues' Benevento said. As a result, the Florida Blues is now offering customers a Platform for Affordable Choices, which comprises a series of options with similarities to previous HMO offerings, as well as PPO products, that are designed to best fit the individual's family and personal needs.

### Equal Satisfaction

According to a recent Consumer Reports survey, HMO respondents were just as satisfied with their health plan as those in PPOs, even when asked about their choice of doctors and care from physicians. Overall, 57% of respondents in PPO and 55% in HMOs said they were highly satisfied with their managed-care plan.

"While we have all heard the horror stories about HMOs, consumer-satisfaction scores still support that customers with HMOs are very satisfied with their coverage, just as they are with their PPO plans," said Rita Costello, senior vice president of strategic marketing and analysis for CareFirst Blue Cross Blue Shield.

---

*"Consumer-satisfaction scores still support that customers with HMOs are very satisfied with their coverage."*—**Rita Costello, CareFirst Blue Cross Blue Shield**

---

PPO satisfaction lies more with service, such as claims processing and administrative functions, while HMO satisfaction is more centered on access to care, including navigating referral processes and getting to see physicians, said Blue Shield of California's Wood.

"HMO enrollment is likely to continue to decline, but some people—those who like the more paternalistic approach of HMO—will still seek them out, and those consumers looking for flexibility, control and choice will seek out PPOs," said Katz of WellPoint. Both will be able to find what they're looking for, and both will find an equal level of satisfaction, he added.

Some insurers,. however, believe consumers' satisfaction with PPOs is continuing to come out ahead of HMOs. "Satifactiona is much greater in PPO-type plans because consumers are more involved and aware of what's going on with their care," said Linde of Destiny Health.

### Continued Winner?

While some insurers believe the cycle may eventually lead to a resurgence for HMOs, most are confident that the next few years will remain the "decade of the PPO."

"I wouldn't be surprised to see HMOs gain some market share in the future as the issue of cost continues to escalate and makes more restrictive plans attractive again," said Dr. Mark Banks, president and CEO of Blue Cross Blue Shield of Minnesota. But the flexibility and choices of PPOs will keep them growing for quite some time, he added.

"PPOs are definitely here to stay," said Watson Wyatt'ss Abbott, who believes consumers' continued interest in a nongatekeeper-type approach, like a PPO or more open-access type products, will bolster PPOs' stronghold as a leader in health plan.

"I think consumers' messages have come across loud and clear—they want freedom of choice—and PPOs will continue to grow and prosper in offering them that choice," said Humana's Bierbower.

PPOs will likely see changes, however, including the possibility of becoming more highly regionalized, and not state specific, said CareFirst's Costello. In addition, she said the next-generation PPO will be more select than today's models. "It won't just be about cost, but also about Performance, which in the end equates to customers satisfaction and positive outcome."

# Medical Savings Account: The Health Insurance Secret[5]

BY STEVE PIELACHA
*INSIDE TUSCON BUSINESS*, FEBRUARY 18–24, 2002

Medical Savings Accounts are the last hope we have to control sky-rocketing health insurance premiums. Local small businesses are seeing rate increases of 20 percent, 30 percent, 40 percent and even higher.

When Congress passed Medical Savings Accounts into law in 1997, it was a pilot project to see if the concept would work. The law allowed insurance companies to offer MSAs in conjunction with "qualifying" large deductible major medical policies to the self-employed and companies with fewer than 50 employees.

The concept would be available to the first 750,000 people in entire nation. To date, fewer than 100,000 people have taken advantage of the opportunity to cut their health insurance premium costs. Of the 100,000 people signed up, approximately 42 percent were previously uninsured because they could either not afford the HMO or did not want to spend money on something they would not use.

With the typical HMO or PPO plan, we send the insurance company a check every month for medical care. On top of the premium, there are co-pays with the HMOs and deductibles and co-insurance with the PPOs. If you have low claims or no claims one year, do they send you a refund check? Of course they don't. They keep it and call it profit.

One Problem with the managed care model is the mentality that we are spending someone else's money . . . "it's only it $20 doctor visit." That may explain why doctors have to see 40 or 50 patients a day.

The other problem with managed care is it seems the HMOs are more conccerned with managing your money than they are with managing your care.

With the MSA concept, you take the money you would ordinarily give the HMO or insurance company and divide it in two parts. Part one, you would buy a large deductible major medical policy to cover you for the big bills. The choices of deductibles allowed by federal law are $1,650 or $2,500 for a single person and $3,300 or $4,950 for a family. The family deductible is combined for the entire family and not per person. The monthly cost for the family $4,950 deductible is about half the cost of the typical HMO.

---

Part two of the MSA concept is the savings account itself. The money you save every month because you bought the large deductible policy can then be put in the MSA, Deposits to this account are 100 percent tax deductible up to certain limits. Individuals can deposit up to 65 percent of the deductible every year and families can deposit up to 75 percent of the deductible. This is the account you would use for routine doctor visits, dental, vision, prescriptions and even "alternative therapies."

If you have an HMO, the charges for dental, vision and alternative therapies are typically paid for out of pocket.

The MSA concept now makes you the consumer of medical care because you spend your money out of your MSA. You decide if you want to use the money for a $49 pair of glasses or a $490 pair of glasses. What you don't spend is yours to keep. There is a misconception floating around that the drawback to the MSA is that what you don't spend by the end of the year is forfeited. That is simply not true. The money grows tax deferred until retirement. This gives people the incentive to shop for health care the way they shop for anything else. Because now it is their money they are spending.

Most polls relating to health care in this country show that most Americans want control and choices when it comes to their health. What better way to take control of your health care dollars than with a high-deductible major medical policy combined with a 100 percent tax-deductible savings account

HMOs used to be the cheapest way to buy health care coverage. But when it comes to your health, do you really want the cheapest or the best coverage you can get for the buck? The MSA concept is worth looking into especially if you are relatively healthy and are self-employed or own a small business.

It's too bad the health insurance industry has kept this a secret. But now that I think about it, I guess they like getting all of your money every month instead of half of it.

# Bridge over Troubled Waters[6]

By Rudy M. Yandrick
*HR Magazine*, October, 2000

Proponents say critical illness insurance fills a need not met by other types of employer-sponsored insurance benefits.

The life of Jimmy Zee, corporate director for Edison, N.J.-based Joule Industrial Contractors, was turned upside down in 1997 when his daughter Valari was diagnosed with an aggressive and rare form of leukemia that required an immediate bone marrow transplant.

"Every day, my wife and I had to make decisions affecting whether my daughter lived or died," he recalls.

As it turns out, Zee had made one of the most important decisions months earlier, when he began offering a cancer expense insurance policy to Joule employees as a voluntary benefit in the company's flexible spending plan. That policy, which he purchased for his family, financed a three-month leave from work (and a six-month leave for his wife from her job) to tend to his daughter's needs during chemotherapy and isolation. The time that it afforded Zee and his wife may have helped save Valari's life.

The cancer-expense plan that Zee purchased is a forerunner of a new type of coverage—critical illness insurance (CII)—that only recently has been introduced in the United States. Nearly all CII plans cover cancer, heart attack, stroke, kidney failure and major organ transplant, although some policies cover far more.

The concept is simple: CII pays for extraneous, usually non-medical, expenses incurred during an episode of major illness, often in a single lump-sum payment. In Zee's case, he received several payouts from his insurer totaling $48,000—money to spend as he saw fit with no strings attached. "I never needed to worry about how I would pay my mortgage if I took off the time from work," he says, a financial reality that many unprotected people do not escape. According to the U.S. Department of Housing and Urban Development, half of all fore-closures on private homes are due to serious illness.

CII is commonly viewed as stopgap coverage to life, medical or disability plans. Due partly to the increasing frequency with which patients survive their illnesses, CII is rapidly gaining popularity in the United States, as it already has done in South Africa, the United Kingdom, Japan and Canada.

---

6. Reprinted with the permission of *HR Magazine*, published by the Society for Human Resource Management, Alexandria, VA.

"People wanted to protect their family members in the event that they die, but they started to ask about how they would meet their bills in the event that they live," says Warren Steele, vice president of marketing for AFLAC, through which Zee purchased his coverage.

Mortality tables justify this concern. For example, the first-year survival rates for heart attack patients increased from 45 percent in 1950 to 70 percent in 1992, from 30 percent to 54 percent for cancer sufferers, and from 24 percent to 73 percent for stroke victims.

But survival creates a financial hardship for families. Life insurance pays only upon death, disability insurance pays only a portion of income in case of total disability, and long-term care reimburses only custodial care services. Meanwhile, studies show that two-thirds of critical illness expenses are non-medical.

And because many health plans severely restrict payments for out-of-network health care, families can be left to foot huge medical bills, especially with conditions that require continuous care. "If someone wants to go to the Mayo Clinic or Sloan Kettering for treatment, their medical plans might fall short of covering the costs," says Kenneth Smith, product manager of supplemental health insurance for Mutual of Omaha. "What's more, when they make the trip, they are accompanied by family or friends in the vast majority of cases. Critical illness insurance helps to cushion the expenses."

## Finding Its Niche

CII is so new that health care consumers are hard pressed to find comparable insurance products. "If there is a direct analogy," says Stacey L. Rollings, assistant vice president of marketing and product engineering for Pacific Life & Annuity in Fountain Valley, Calif., "it is accidental death and dismemberment coverage," which pays out a lump sum for loss of use of eyes, limbs, etc. "The difference is, AD&D is more injury-focused, while CII is more disease-focused."

The profusion in employee benefits also is abetting CII's popularity. To HR managers, it can be an attractive option to the company benefit plan. "There are so many different employee interests and family situations today," says Jerome Mattern, SPHR, HR manager for Quebecor World in St. Cloud, Minn., and chair of the Society for Human Resource Management's Compensation and Benefits Committee. "HR managers are being very responsive to employees by providing them with more options." CII might be particularly appealing to a young, two-career couple interested in protecting their assets for only a few premium dollars, he explains.

Built-in cost control is another incentive. "Compared with major medical insurance, you are getting a fixed benefit," says Mutual of Omaha's Smith. "You don't have [medical] inflation to deal with"—

a cost increase that has outpaced consumer inflation over the last 20 years. " I'm not aware of a single carrier that has raised rates so far."

### What Is a Critical Illness?

Two potential problems for CII policyholders are limits in the number of illnesses covered and restrictive definitions of individual illnesses, which potentially could preclude a payout. HR managers considering a CII policy for their employees should ensure that at least the five primary critical illnesses are covered.

Additional illnesses or conditions may include coma, paralysis, coronary surgery, bypass and others.

In the United Kingdom, some carriers cover as many as 30 illnesses and other conditions, greatly complicating the policies for both insurers and beneficiaries. In the 1980s, covered conditions were stacked upon one another by life insurers as customer enticements in a derby for new business. Among the conditions commonly covered are AIDS/HIV, bacterial meningitis, aplastic anemia, benign brain tumor, blindness and deafness.

> *Having the benefit of overseas markets as pilot sites, U.S. insurers are taking steps to limit their coverage to definable illnesses.*

According to Roger Edwards, product marketing manager for Scottish Provident UK, "One insurer would cover eight illnesses and the next would cover 10, and so forth, until everybody realized they were creating a lot of confusion, but not necessarily selling any more policies. Since then, we've turned our focus to education about the benefits of CII coverage and have found a more receptive audience."

Another potential problem as more conditions are added is the increased potential for disputes over whether a policyholder's particular illness meets the insurer's criteria. Having the benefit of overseas markets as pilot sites, U.S. insurers are taking steps to limit their coverage to definable illnesses. "We don't cover blindness because there are varying degrees of impairment, such as 70 percent versus 100 percent," says AFLAC's Steele. "The degree for other conditions such as coma is based on time. An insurer may define coma based on a vegetative state lasting at least seven days, while another may define it as at least 14."

### Continental Divide

In the United Kingdom, CII has been growing since the mid-1980s as supplemental life insurance. According to Swiss Re Life, which conducts an annual survey of life and pension plans, new policy sales exceeded 750,000 in 1999, a 12.8 percent increase over 1998. Sales of new individual CII policies as a percentage of regular premium life policy sales have steadily increased from 4.9 percent of sales in 1992 to 24.5 percent last year. (No such industry statistics are yet available in the U.S.)

By contrast, in the United States, CII is sold more often as a stand alone supplemental health insurance product than as a life insurance rider, according to Tony Boston, a Devon, U.K.-based actuarial consultant to both U.S. and British companies. This is the likely result of consumer angst over restrictive managed care practices that limit treatment options and payments, which may leave the patient to foot more of the bill for expensive medical treatment.

Additionally, "a payment from a stand-alone CII policy is universally agreed to be tax-free, while the IRS has not yet ruled on the tax status of a payment from a rider which 'accelerates' part of the underlying face amount," explains Boston.

Employers and policyholders will find CII to be a modest additional expense compared to medical insurance, whether it is purchased as a standalone health product or as a life insurance rider. However, premiums will vary depending on the illnesses covered, dollar value of the plan, and policyholder age and health habits, especially smoking.

*Critics variously cite CII as a needless frill or a money- making scheme for insurers.*

"CII premiums run about two to two-and-a-half times as much as life insurance, although there's no hard-and-fast formula," says Pacific Life & Annuity's Rollings. "For the average worker, coverage might be $20 to $25 a month."

CII premiums vary widely, though. For example, a nonsmoking 25-year-old may pay less than $50 per year on a $5,000 policy, while a 60-year-old smoker can expect to pay almost $4,000 a year on a $100,000 policy. With respect to the amount of CII coverage to purchase, Smith offers this rule of thumb: "a person should be able to replace 12 months of income."

Many plans provide a lump-sum payout, then terminate. Others pay out incrementally based on initial diagnosis, first treatment and recurrences. There may be a 30-day waiting period following initial diagnosis, the rationale being that if the person does not survive the 30 days, their life insurance plan will be activated for survivors. In the meantime, though, it can create financial instability during a period of personal turmoil.

**Read the Fine Print**

Critics variously cite CII as a needless frill or a moneymaking scheme for insurers. According to Gail Shearer, director of health policy analysis for the Consumers Union, "the bottom line here is 'let the buyer beware.' If a critical illness occurs, you might get some cash. At worst, focusing on critical illness coverage can divert consumers' attention from badly needed comprehensive [health care] coverage."

Before offering CII coverage for employees, an HR manager should consider:

- Whether the money could be better spent improving the company's medical policy by lowering deductibles, lowering coinsurance, reducing employee-paid premiums or providing a greater choice of providers.

- What the definitions of the illnesses are. This is pivotal in determining whether a person with a health condition qualifies for a payout.

- Whether family members can be added, and what the costs are.

- Whether the policy terminates after it is cashed out following first occurrence of a critical illness.

- Whether the CII policy qualifies as a Section 125 benefit, which enables the beneficiary to pay for the plan using pre-tax dollars. Currently, CII plans that pay a lump sum based on diagnosis instead of treatment are not eligible, since they are not considered a medical benefit.

- Whether state departments of insurance have issued a cautionary statement about a particular company or CII policy.

- What an insurer's ratio of payouts to total premiums, or loss ratio, is.

- Whether the policy terminates at a certain age, such as 65 or 70.

An inherent risk of CII coverage, admit both proponents and opponents, is the temptation to view it as a lottery: get sick, quit work and be financially independent. One way that a policy can preclude such a loser-take-all scheme is by stretching out the payments, rather than issuing a single lump sum. Another may be to link CII with wellness plans intended to prevent the very illnesses that trigger the coverage's payouts. In this way, by detecting a minor health condition for which there is no CII benefit, a major, payable condition could be averted later on.

"With hypertension or angina, for example, a policyholder diagnosed with one of these will be given a treatment plan of diet and exercise. This may well mean that the patient will not suffer from a heart attack later," says Boston. Although this theory remains to be proven, he predicts that it will break new ground for insurance actuaries in the coming years.

When the pros and cons are considered, it is hard to deny that CII can be a life raft when critical illness disrupts a family's life.

In Jimmy Zee's case, the critical illness insurance bought another commodity for him and his wife: time. Valari was treated as part of a bone marrow transplant group at a children's hospital. The Zees were the only parents with the luxury of staying with their daughter—the only member of her patient group to survive—throughout her intensive care.

All of the other children's parents had work duties to attend to, and often were unable to see their children in their final moments. Says Zee, "As I have talked since then with the other parents, that is the one thing they tell me they wish they had: more time at the end."

# The Bill for Rights[7]

By Carl E. Schneider
*Hastings Center Report*, January–February 2002

Where today is legislative ingenuity lavished more bountifully than on the titles of statutes? And where has that ingenuity been better exercised than in the name "patients' bill of rights"? Do not our dearest liberties flow from the Bill of Rights? And who more deserves similar protection than patients in the hands of an angry Managed Care Organization? And behold, both Democrats and Republicans, both President Clinton and President Bush, have summoned us to arms. The patients' bill of rights is an idea whose time has seemed to have come for several years, and only conflicts among the numerous proposals and 11 September have postponed the apparently inevitable.

The impetus for legislation is irresistible. Its name is managed care. American medicine has moved from cottage industry to bureaucratic behemoth with imposing and implacable speed. Ought not combinations of great size—malefactors of great wealth—be regulated, especially when their services can literally be vital? What is more, cost containment with bite, once a fantasy, is becoming a reality. When medical bureaucracies are commanded to conserve resources, they in turn drive physicians into an ethically tense position—serving both the god of patients' welfare and the Mammon of MCO profits. Ought not government police that conflict of interest?

And where are the police when we need them? Preempted. Our federal system confides government supervision of medicine to the states. However, most people obtain medical insurance from their employers' benefits plans. In 1974, the federal government, concerned about the safety of employers' pensions, enacted the Employee Retirement Income Security Act to safeguard them. To protect ERISA's strictures, that statute "supersede[s] any and all State laws insofar as they may now or hereafter relate to any employee benefit, plan." Although ERISA was primarily aimed at pensions, it covers employee benefits generally, including medical benefits. Thus while states may continue to make individual doctors liable for medical wrongs like malpractice, various other kinds of MCO activities—and not least their cost-control programs—may escape the states' regulation, at least insofar as those programs are part of an employee benefit plan. (I say "may" because the extent to which ERISA preempts state regulation of MCOs remains grossly uncertain even after the Supreme Court's recent encounter with that question in *Pegram v. Herdrich*.[1]) And while the federal government has not been inactive, neither has it acted systematically.

The case I have so far sketched for a patients' bill of rights is circumstantial: MCOs must want to economize, they must pressure doctors to do so, doctors must acquiesce, this must injure patients, and thus patients must be endowed with rights. Arguments for regulating managed care are not, however, solely circumstantial; they are also anecdotal. What journalist trying to make the dull vivid, what politician trying to make duty plain, could resist the anecdotes lobbyists luridly spread before them? In their canonical form, these anecdotes tell of someone dying of a dreadful disease, someone without hope unless a bureaucracy will let doctors do their jobs and will pay for a "cutting-edge" treatment. These anecdotes are supplemented by stories that resonate with us all about bureaucratic intrigue, incompetence, and insolence.

---

### *Arguments for regulating managed care are not . . . solely circumstantial; they are also anecdotal.*

---

So there is a circumstantial and anecdotal case for regulation. And that case has become the case for a patients' bill of rights. Versions of that device throng like leaves in Vallombrosa and change about is frequently, so generalization is hazardous. Politically prominent versions, however, have attempted—often in ambitious and elaborate ways—to establish procedures MCOs must use in utilization reviews, to require appeals outside the MCO of denials of treatment, to specify what services MCOs must provide, to state what information MCOs must and must not furnish, to restrict MCOs from using incentive systems to influence doctors' decisions, to extend patients' ability to sue their MCOs, and on and on.

Well, who could object to any of this? In a later column I will examine specific provisions that are actually enacted or seem about to be. Here I will suggest seven questions we should ask before succumbing to the conventional wisdom about "the need for a strong patients' bill of rights," as conventional wisdom's fount, the *New York Times* editorial page put it.[2]

First, how convincing is the evidence that legislation is necessary? Circumstantial evidence and anecdotes are pitiful bases for public policy, but they may be irresistible when they confirm what seems obvious. Nevertheless, it is wise to doubt the obvious, and there are especially provoking reasons to do so here. For example, it is widely assumed that MCOs' efforts to economize must mean that they offer worse care than their alternatives. Yet "[o]verall, the evidence . . . does not support the premise that managed care has lowered the effectiveness of care."[3] It is also widely assumed, and doctors widely insist, that MCOs rob physicians of time with patients. Yet during the period in which MCOs have proliferated, the time doctors spend with patients has actually increased.[4]

> *Patients' bills of rights are largely directed against the aspects of managed care that have helped tame costs.*

Second, what are the goals of a patient' bill of rights? To make health care more efficient? More accountable? Fairer? Cheaper? Better? These are only a few of the possible goals. And they are all worthy goals, but a statute that serves one often disserves others. If we simply ask whether a bill of rights promotes one desirable end, we may overlook the way it interferes with others.

Third, will a patients' bill of rights accomplish its goals? Law often frustrates its makers, and the history of bioethical legal reform has been the history of humiliation. Why expect a bill of rights to do better? For example, bills of rights unimaginatively attempt to bring "due process" to the MCO. In other areas, due process solutions repeatedly go unutilized by the people they intend to benefit. A recent survey of research on the effects of MCOs finds that "sick enrollees who are poor or elderly fare worse in HMOs."[5] But such patients are exactly the people least likely to be aggressive enough to wring results from due process rights. Put it this way: is the only cure for the ills of bureaucracy more bureaucracy?

Fourth, *cui bono*—who benefits? Patients' bills of rights are piously described as serving patients. But doctors' groups have been instrumental in framing and promoting many of them. "The voice is Jacob's voice, but the hands are the hands of Esau." Have doctors' groups again succumbed to the temptation of advocating legislation that benefits the profession more than the patient? Bioethicists have written for years about the "abject" relationship of patient to doctor. MCOs are the only countervailing force on the horizon. In short, if medical costs are to be cabined and medical care to be improved, doctors' power will need to be constrained, not institutionalized under the banner of patients' rights.

Fifth, in a medical world in turbulent change, are these the rules we want to enact into legislation that will be hard to alter? Managed care has gone from marginal to predominant in hardly more than a decade, and it continues to develop tumultuously. A bill of rights attempts to enshrine timeless principles. Are these they? For instance, even as Congress debates mandating cumbersome procedures for utilization reviews, at least one prominent MCO has "decided to abandon utilization review mechanisms due to their cost and the relatively small number of recommended treatments that were found to be inappropriate."[6]

Sixth, is the legislation so harmless that nothing can be lost by enacting it? If bills of rights simply ask MCOs to do what is plainly right, why not pass one? Here, we must remember what brought us to MCOs—namely, the struggle to subdue health care costs. Governmental efforts were feeble and failed. Employers acted by promoting MCOs. They seem to have won a battle, but the war remains perilously in doubt. Patients' bills of rights are largely directed against the aspects of managed care that have helped tame costs. Few argue that we should devote more of our GDP to health care. Employers yearn to control health care costs. Employees, when given a choice about whether to buy mom extensive health insurance or to spend their money elsewhere, repeatedly choose the latter, so that patients' bills of rights seem likely to impose on people insurance more expensive than they would choose to buy for themselves. Small wonder, then, that support for bills of rights plummets when their costs are described. And small wonder that while Congress congratulates itself for imposing a bill of rights on private MCOs, it hesitates to inflict one on federal programs.

Seventh, is a patients' bill of rights where we should spend scarce reformist energies? Congress has repeatedly failed to formulate cogent health policy, and it has tried only sporadically. Such moments ought not be wasted. Let me make the point a challenge: Should a country in which more than 40 million people lack health insurance expend limited human and legislative resources to make medical care more expensive—but not necessarily better—for those who already have it?

These seven questions about patients' bills of rights have been skeptical. But they are the same questions we should ask about any health care legislation. And one reasonable inference from them is that many kinds of proposals ought to be considered. Law's arsenal enjoys various weapons. One, for example, is the law of contract. It might seek to build on the market's energy and creativity in devising managed care but to structure the market to better reflect what patients want. Another weapon is the law of tort. Perhaps much can be gained by shifting malpractice liability from individual doctors to MCOs and hospitals. Yet another weapon is to assign government agencies regulatory authority, an approach that seems most successful when the agency seeks less to write and enforce its own rules than to stimulate an industry to intelligent and aggressive self-regulation. But, surely, before seizing any weapon, systematic inquiry into its costs and its benefits is essential.

## References

1.  530 U.S. 211 (2000).
2.  "Curing the Patients' Bill Rights," *New York Times* 4 September 2001.

3.  F.J. Hellinger. "The Effect of Managed Care on Quality: A Review of Recent Evidence," *Archives of Internal Medicine* 158 (1998): 833–841, at 840.

4.  D. Mechanic and D.D. McAlpine, "'Fifteen Minutes of Fame': Reflections on the Uses of Health Research, the Media, Pundits, and the Spin," *Health Affairs* 20 (2001): 211–215.

5.  Hellinger, "The Effects of Managed Care on Quality."

6.  G.B. Agrawal, "Resuscitating Professionalism: Self-Regulation in the Medical Marketplace," *Missouri Law Review* 66 (201): 341–411, at 356, n. 74.

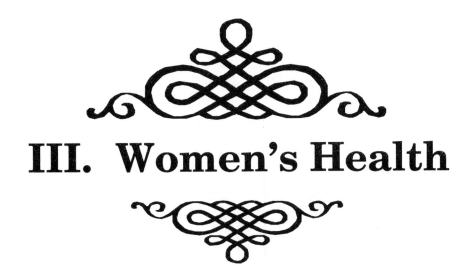

# III.  Women's Health

# Editor's Introduction

For years, doctors thought that the top health concerns and diseases that affected men were the same ones that afflicted women. Because of this misconception, women often did not receive accurate medical advice or information. Although doctors have come to realize that women manifest different symptoms from men for the same illnesses, women are still not fully informed about the diseases that should concern them most. Chapter 3 deals exclusively with women's health issues and the need for women to be better educated about their bodies to maintain good health.

Although the health of American women has improved in the last decade, it still does not meet the nation's standards. "Women's State Health Rankings Improve Slightly" compares a 2000 report on women's health to a 2001 report. It discusses areas in which improvements are still needed by each state, such as in the diagnosis and treatment of diabetes and heart disease, as well as in the number of women with health insurance.

The next article in this section focuses on the leading cause of death among women in the United States: heart disease. At one time, it was believed that women were not prone to heart attacks. Even today, symptoms are often misdiagnosed in women, and heart attacks go untreated or undetected. "Heart Disease and Women: Are You at Risk," discusses what heart disease and stroke are, the risk factors, and what can be done to prevent or minimize those risks.

Termed "the whispering killer," ovarian cancer is even more difficult to detect in women than heart disease. Its symptoms are not outwardly apparent and can resemble those of other, more innocuous conditions, often causing doctors to misdiagnose it. Marcia Mattson reports on one woman's first-hand experience fighting ovarian cancer in "The Quiet Enemy." From descriptions of her symptoms to her diagnosis and treatment, this article personalizes the struggle against ovarian cancer. Mattson also discusses steps doctors should take to rule out its presence in their patients.

Unlike heart disease and ovarian cancer, breast cancer is often caught early by doctors in women who receive yearly mammograms and perform breast self-examinations. As Donald D. Hensrud explains in "A Woman's Greatest Fear," many women know that their chances of developing breast cancer increase when a close relative is diagnosed with it. Many others, however, do not realize that 75% of breast cancer cases occur in women who are not obviously at risk. Hensrud looks at the risk factors involved, discusses how women should check for breast cancer, and stresses the importance of mammograms. An accompanying sidebar dispels some common myths about the disease.

Eating disorders are another condition that primarily, though not exclusively, affects females. Roughly 50,000 Americans will die this year from eating disorders, which afflict between 5 and 10 million women, putting them at a higher risk for heart disease, kidney failure, osteoporosis, and death. While there are several theories as to why women develop eating disorders, Jennifer Pirtle examines the notion that these problems could be genetically determined. In her article "Why Don't They Just Eat?" Pirtle looks at one girl's ultimately successful struggle with anorexia nervosa.

At some point in their lifetimes, all women will go through menopause, making it an important subject to include in this chapter. Though different women will experience it at different ages, menopausal symptoms vary from hot flashes to an increased risk of breast cancer. In her article "The Menopause Decision," Dahpna Caperonis looks at two womens' struggles with menopause and their experiences trying to treat it. Caparonis describes the different symptoms they experienced while using both natural herbal remedies and traditional hormone replacements, the side effects of each, and what types of therapies ultimately worked best for them.

# Women's State Health Rankings Improve Slightly[1]

*NATION'S HEALTH*, FEBRUARY 2002

A few states have made inroads in improving women's health, but progress nationwide is still unsatisfactory, according to a recent report.

Too many women continue to be uninsured, live in poverty, be overweight and have high blood pressure, diabetes and osteoporosis, according to the report, "Making the Grade on Women's Health: A National and State-by-State Report Card 2001."

"It's time—past time—for bold action at both the state and federal levels," said Regan E. Ralph, JD, vice president of health and reproductive rights at the National Women's Law Center. "In no state do women enjoy satisfactory health status based on the nation's own standards."

The report, a follow-up to the first such report card in 2000, was released in December by the National Women's Law Center, the Oregon Health and Science University and Focus on Health and Leadership for Women at the University of Pennsylvania School of Medicine.

The rankings were based on health status and health policy indicators that were set by Healthy People goals. The states were given grades of "satisfactory," "unsatisfactory-plus," "unsatisfactory" or "fail."

Only one state, Louisiana, received a failing grade in 2001, compared to eight states and the District of Columbia in 2000, but, for the second year, no state received a "satisfactory" grade.

The findings did, however, show some progress: Twelve states strengthened safety net services, while 11 gave patients the right to demand external review of managed care decisions. Fifteen states and the District of Columbia improved coverage for medications for low-income people not eligible for Medicaid.

However, only four states made any progress in reducing the number of uninsured women, and four states improved their Medicaid coverage for single parents.

There was only one area in which all 50 states and the District of Columbia met the national benchmark: the percentage of women age 50 and older who receive mammograms. In 2000 and 2001,

1. Article from *The Nation's Health* February 2002. Copyright © American Public Health Association. Reprinted with permission.

there were eight areas in which every state and the District of Columbia fell below the national benchmark, including uninsured women, overweight, diabetes and the wage gap.

The report includes a special section on cardiovascular disease, pointing out that cardiovascular disease is the leading killer of women in the United States.

"A close look at women and cardiovascular disease reveals many of the problems that plague women throughout our health care system—inadequate research and data collection, a failure to understand how the disease affects women, a lack of preventive services and poor health care once the disease strikes," said Michelle Berlin, MD, MPH, associate professor at Oregon.

Women are more likely than men to delay seeking care after the onset of heart attack symptoms and to suffer a second heart attack within six years of the first, Berlin said.

However, women are less likely than men to have their heart attack symptoms recognized by a doctor, to receive counseling on risk factors or to be enrolled in rehabilitation programs after a heart attack, she said.

The country as a whole received a failing grade on key indicators related to cardiovascular disease: smoking, overweight, physical inactivity, poor nutrition and high blood pressure.

# Heart Disease and Women: Are You At Risk?[2]

By National Heart, Lung, and Blood Institute
*WWW.NHLBI.NIH.GOV*, August 1998

Heart disease is a woman's concern. Every woman's concern. One in ten American women 45 to 64 years of age has some form of heart disease, and this increases to one in four women over 65. Heart disease is the number one killer of American women. In addition, 2 million women have had a stroke, and 93,000 women die of stroke each year.

This fact sheet tells you what kinds of habits and health conditions increase the chances of developing these diseases—and what you can do to keep your heart healthy.

## What Are These Diseases?

Both heart disease and stroke are known as cardiovascular diseases, which are disorders of the heart and blood vessel system. Coronary heart disease—the main subject of this fact sheet—is a disease of the blood vessels of the heart, known as "coronary arteries." Coronary heart disease causes chest pain (angina) and heart attacks. Blood brings oxygen and nutrients to the heart. When too little blood flows to the heart, angina results. When the blood flow is critically reduced, a heart attack occurs. A lack of blood flow to the brain or, in some cases, bleeding in the brain causes a stroke. Some other cardiovascular diseases are high blood pressure and rheumatic heart disease.

## Who Gets Cardiovascular Diseases?

Some women have more "risk factors" for cardiovascular diseases than others. Risk factors are habits or traits that make a person more likely to develop a disease. Some risk factors for heart-related problems cannot be changed, but many others can be.

The major risk factors for cardiovascular disease that you can do something about are cigarette smoking, high blood pressure, high blood cholesterol, overweight, and physical inactivity. Other risk factors, such as diabetes, also are conditions you have some control over. Even just one risk factor will raise your chances of having

2. Article by U.S. Department of Health and Human Services; Public Health Service, National Institutes of Health, National Heart, Lung, and Blood Institute. NIH Publication No. 98-3654. Originally printed 1995. Revised August 1998.

heart-related problems. But the more risk factors you have, the more likely you are to develop cardiovascular diseases—and the more concerned you should be about protecting your heart health.

# Major Risk Factors

## Smoking

Smoking by women in the United States causes one and a half times as many deaths from heart disease as from lung cancer. If you smoke, you are two to six times more likely to suffer a heart attack than a nonsmoking woman, and the risk increases with the number of cigarettes you smoke each day. Smoking also boosts the risk of stroke.

> ### Heart Disease Risk Factors
>
> Risk factors are habits or traits that make a person more likely to develop a disease. Many of those for heart disease can be controlled. These include:
> - Cigarette smoking
> - High blood pressure
> - High blood cholesterol
> - Overweight
> - Physical inactivity
> - Diabetes
>
> The more risk factors you have, the greater your risk. So take action—take control!

Cardiovascular diseases are not the only health risks connected to smoking. Women who smoke are much more likely to develop lung cancer than nonsmoking women. Cigarette smoking is also linked with cancers of the mouth, larynx, esophagus, urinary tract, kidney, pancreas, and cervix. Smokers also are more likely to develop other kinds of lung problems, including bronchitis and emphysema.

Smoking during pregnancy is also linked to a number of problems. They include bleeding, miscarriage, premature delivery, lower birth weight, stillbirth, and sudden infant death syndrome, or "crib death." Also, young children who breathe in a parent's cigarette smoke have more lung and ear infections.

There is simply no safe way to smoke. Although low-tar and low-nicotine cigarettes may reduce the lung cancer risk somewhat, they do not lessen the risks of heart diseases or other smoking-related diseases. The only safe and healthful course is not to smoke at all.

## High Blood Pressure

High blood pressure, also known as hypertension, is another major risk factor for coronary heart disease and the most important risk factor for stroke and heart failure. Heart failure is a severe condition in which the heart cannot adequately supply the body with blood. High blood pressure causes three of every five cases of heart failure in women. High blood pressure also boosts the chances of developing kidney disease and blindness.

Older women have a higher risk of high blood pressure, with more than half of all women over age 55 suffering from this condition. High blood pressure is more common and more severe in African-American women than it is in white women. Using birth control pills can contribute to high blood pressure in some women.)

While all women can and should take steps to prevent or control high blood pressure, it is especially important for women who have heart disease to do so. When blood pressure is lowered, the heart does not work as hard. Women who have had a heart attack are less likely to have another if they reduce their high blood pressure.

> ### Remember: Get Your Blood Pressure Checked
>
> The higher your blood pressure, the greater your risk for coronary heart disease. If your blood pressure is above 140/90 mmHg, you should consult your doctor at once. Even if your blood pressure is normal, you can lower it—and reduce your risk for coronary artery disease.
>
> Talk to your doctor to discuss the steps you should take to keep your blood pressure at a healthy level.

What is blood pressure—and when is it high? Blood pressure is the amount of force exerted by the blood against the walls of the arteries. Everyone has to have some blood pressure, so that blood can get to the body's organs and muscles. Usually, blood pressure is expressed as two numbers, such as 120/80 mmHg (millimeters of mercury). Depending on your activities, blood pressure may rise or fall in the course of a day. Blood pressure is considered high when it stays above 140/90 mmHg over a period of time.

However, the harmful effects of elevated blood pressure do not begin at the 140/90 mmHg mark—even blood pressures slightly under that can increase your risk of heart disease and stroke. Also, both numbers are important to your health. Many older Americans, for example, have a form of high blood pressure known as "isolated systolic hypertension" (ISH). This occurs when the systolic pressure (the top number) is high but the diastolic pressure (the bottom number) is normal. This too, if not controlled, increases the risk of heart attack and stroke.

High blood pressure is called the "silent killer" because most people who have it do not feel sick. That means it is important to have it checked regularly. Because blood pressure changes often, your doctor or other health professional should check it on several different days before deciding if your blood pressure is too high.

Although high blood pressure can rarely be cured, it can be controlled with proper treatment. If your blood pressure is not too high, you may be able to control it entirely through weight loss if you are overweight, regular physical activity, and cutting down on alcohol and salt and sodium. (Sodium is an ingredient in salt that is found in many packaged foods, carbonated beverages, baking soda, and some antacids.

It may also help to eat more fruits and vegetables and low fat or nonfat dairy products that supply plenty of potassium, magnesium, fiber, and calcium. Eating foods rich in potassium, in particular, seems to prevent high blood pressure.

However, if your blood pressure remains high, your doctor may prescribe medicine in addition to the above changes, especially if you already have heart disease. The amount of medicine you take may be gradually reduced, especially if you are successful with the changes you make in your lifestyle.

A reminder: Be sure to take a blood pressure medication exactly as your doctor has prescribed it. Blood pressure medicine must be taken in the right amounts and at the right times in order to work properly.

During pregnancy, some women develop high blood pressure for the first time. Other women who already have high blood pressure may find that it gets worse during pregnancy. If untreated, these conditions can be life-threatening to both mother and baby. Since

---

### BLOOD PRESSURE CATEGORIES IN WOMEN (18 YEARS AND OLDER)*

Blood pressure is shown as two numbers—the systolic pressure as the heart is beating and the diastolic pressure between heartbeats. Both numbers are important.

**Blood Pressure Level in mmHg**

| Category | Systolic | | Diastolic |
|---|---|---|---|
| Optimal** | <120 | and | <80 |
| Normal | <130 | and | <85 |
| High-normal | 130-139 | or | 85-89 |
| Hypertension | | | |
| Stage 1 | 140-159 | or | 90-99 |
| Stage 2 | 160-179 | or | 100-109 |
| Stage 3 | ≥180 | or | ≥110 |

* Not taking antihypertensive drugs and not acutely ill. When systolic and diastolic blood pressures fall into different categories, the higher category determines blood pressure status.

**Optimal blood pressure with respect to cardiovascular risk is <120/<80 mmHg. Unusually low readings should be evaluated for clinical significance.

Source: *The Sixth Report of the Joint National Committee on Detection, Evaluation, and Treatment of High Blood Pressure*, NIH, NHLBI, 1997.

you can feel perfectly normal and still have one of these conditions, be sure to get regular prenatal checkups so your doctor can find and control a possible high blood pressure problem.

Blood pressure tends to get higher as you age. So, even if your blood pressure is normal now, it makes sense to take steps to prevent high blood pressure in the years to come. You will be less likely to develop high blood pressure if you are physically active, maintain a healthy weight, limit your alcohol intake, and cut down on salt and sodium.

## High Blood Cholesterol

High blood cholesterol is another very important risk factor for coronary heart disease that you can do something about. Blood cholesterol levels among women in the United States tend to rise from about the age of 20. But they rise sharply beginning at about age 40 and continue to increase until about age 60. The higher your blood cholesterol level, the higher your heart disease risk.

Today, about a quarter of all American women have blood cholesterol levels high enough to pose a serious risk for heart disease. More than half of the women over age 55 need to lower their blood cholesterol.

While the body needs cholesterol to function normally, it makes enough to meet all of its needs. But too much saturated fat and cholesterol in the food one eats raise the level of cholesterol in the blood. Over a period of years, extra cholesterol and fat in the blood are deposited in the inner walls of the arteries that supply blood to the heart. These deposits make the arteries narrower and narrower. As a result, less blood gets to the heart and the risk of coronary heart disease increases.

---

**BLOOD CHOLESTEROL LEVELS**
**FOR WOMEN WITHOUT HEART DISEASE**

|  | Desirable | Borderline-High | High |
|---|---|---|---|
| **Total cholesterol** | Less than 200 | 200-239 | 240 and above |
| **LDL cholesterol** | Less than 130 | 130-159 | 160 and above |

An HDL cholesterol level of less than 35 is a major risk factor for heart disease.
An HDL level of 60 or higher is protective.

Source: Second Report of the Expert Panel on Detection, and Treatment of High Blood Cholesterol in Adults, NIH, NHLBI, 1993.

---

Cholesterol travels in the blood in packages called lipoproteins. Cholesterol packaged in low density lipoprotein (LDL) is often called "bad" cholesterol, because too much LDL in the blood can lead to cholesterol buildup and blockage in the arteries.

Another type of cholesterol, which is packaged in high density lipoprotein (HDL), is known as "good" cholesterol. That is because HDL helps remove cholesterol from the blood, preventing it from piling up in the arteries.

All women age 20 and older should have their blood cholesterol checked. The following sections describe the steps for managing cholesterol levels for two types of women: those who do not have coronary heart disease, and those who do have coronary heart disease.

### If You Do Not Have Heart Disease

**Getting Your Cholesterol Checked.** Blood cholesterol levels are measured by means of a small blood sample. The blood should be tested for total cholesterol and, if an accurate measurement is available, for HDL cholesterol as well.

**Understanding the Numbers.** A desirable total cholesterol level for adults without heart disease is less than 200 mg/dL (or 200 milligrams per deciliter of blood). A level of 240 mg/dL or above is considered "high" blood cholesterol. But even levels in the "borderline-high" category (200–239 mg/dL) increase the risk of heart disease.

HDL levels are interpreted differently than total cholesterol levels. The lower your HDL level, the higher your heart disease risk. An HDL level of under 35 is a major risk factor for heart disease. A level of 60 or higher is considered protective.

Total and HDL cholesterol are measured first. If these tests show any of the following, your doctor will want to measure your LDL level as well: total cholesterol of 240 mg/dL or above; total cholesterol of 200–239 mg/dL with two or more other risk factors for heart disease; or HDL cholesterol of less than 35 mg/dL.

An LDL level below 130 mg/dL is desirable. LDL levels of 130–159 mg/dL are borderline-high. Levels of 160 mg/dL or above are high. As with total cholesterol, the higher your LDL number, the higher the risk.

**Prevention and Treatment.** If your tests show that your blood cholesterol levels are in the desirable range, keep up the good work! To help keep your levels healthy, it will be important to eat a low saturated fat, low cholesterol diet, engage in regular physical activity, and control your weight.

If your blood cholesterol levels are too high, your doctor may recommend a specific treatment program for you. For most people, cutting back on foods high in saturated fat and cholesterol will lower

LDL cholesterol, which is the main goal of treatment. Regular physical activity and weight loss for overweight persons also will lower blood cholesterol levels.

Losing extra weight, as well as quitting smoking and becoming more physically active, also may help boost your HDL cholesterol level.

If your new diet and other lifestyle changes do not lower your blood cholesterol level enough, your doctor may suggest that you take cholesterol-lowering medications. If you have other risk factors for heart disease, you will need to lower your cholesterol more than someone without risk factors.

### If You Have Heart Disease

Women who have coronary (or "ischemic") heart disease should pay even more attention to their cholesterol levels. An individual with coronary heart disease has a much greater risk of having a future heart attack than a person without heart disease. Whether or not your cholesterol level is elevated, lowering it will greatly reduce your risk of a future heart attack and can actually prolong your life.

**Getting Your Cholesterol Checked.** Since you have heart disease, you will need to have a blood test called a lipoprotein profile. This test will determine not only your total cholesterol and HDL cholesterol levels, but also your levels of LDL cholesterol and another fatty substance called triglycerides.

**Understanding the Numbers.** Your goal should be to have an LDL cholesterol of about 100 mg/dL or less, which is lower than for people who do not have heart disease. Depending on what your LDL level is, your next steps will be the following:

- If your LDL level is 100 mg/dL or less, you do not need to take specific steps to lower your LDL. But you will need to have your level tested again in 1 year. In the meantime, you should closely follow a diet low in saturated fat and cholesterol, maintain a healthy weight, be physically active, and not smoke. You should also follow the specific recommendations of your doctor.

- If your LDL level is higher than 100 mg/dL, you will need a complete physical examination to find out if you have a disease or condition that is raising your cholesterol levels. Then you should take steps to lower your LDL to 100 mg/dL or less: closely follow a low saturated fat, low cholesterol diet, be physically active, lose excess weight, and take cholesterol-lowering medicine, if prescribed. Of course, you also should avoid smoking.

    If, in your doctor's judgment, your LDL level starts out too much higher than the LDL goal of 100 mg/dL or if your LDL level stays too high after lifestyle changes, you will need to take medicine.

## Overweight

Overweight women are much more likely to develop heart-related problems, even if they have no other risk factors. Excess body weight in women is linked with coronary heart disease, stroke, congestive heart failure, and death from heart-related causes. The more overweight you are, the higher your risk for heart disease.

Overweight contributes not only to cardiovascular diseases, but also to other risk factors, including high blood pressure, high blood cholesterol, and diabetes. Fortunately, these conditions often can be controlled with weight loss and regular physical activity.

What is a healthy weight for you? There is no exact answer. Check the "Are You Overweight?" chart to find out if your weight is within the healthy weight range suggested for women of your height. Weights above the suggested ranges are believed to be unhealthy for most people.

*Overweight women are much more likely to develop heart-related problems, even if they have no other risk factors.*

Body shape as well as weight may affect heart health. "Apple-shaped" individuals with extra fat at the waistline may have a higher risk than "pear-shaped" people with heavy hips and thighs. If your waist is nearly as large as, or larger than, the size of your hips, you may have a higher risk for coronary heart disease.

For lasting weight loss, engage in regular, brisk physical activity and eat foods that are low in calories and fat. Do not try to lose more than 1/2 to 1 pound a week.

## Physical Inactivity

Physical inactivity increases the risk of heart disease. It both contributes directly to heart-related problems and increases the chances of developing other risk factors, such as high blood pressure and diabetes.

Physical inactivity is increasing among Americans—especially among women. According to the first-ever *Surgeon General's Report on Physical Activity and Health*, 60 percent of American women do not get the recommended amount of physical activity, while more than 25 percent are not active at all.

Fortunately, it doesn't take a lot of effort to become physically active. The Surgeon General's report and other research conclude that as little as 30 minutes of moderate activity on most, and preferably all, days of the week help protect heart health. Examples of moderate activity are brisk walking or bicycling, raking leaves, or gardening.

If you prefer, you can divide the 30-minute activity into shorter periods of at least 10 minutes each. If you already engage in this level of activity, you can get added benefits by doing even more.

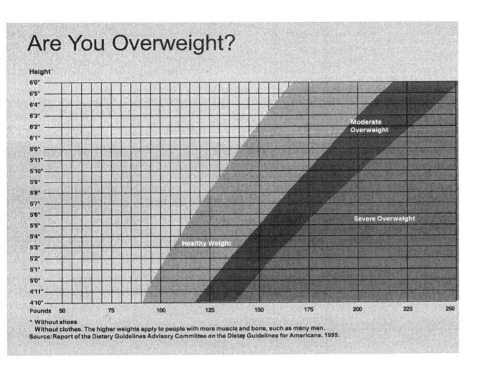

## Are You Overweight?

Height*

6'6"
6'5"
6'4"
6'3"
6'2"                                                          Moderate
6'1"                                                          Overweight
6'0"
5'11"
5'10"
5'9"
5'8"
5'7"
5'6"                                                    Severe Overweight
5'5"
5'4"
5'3"                        Healthy Weight
5'2"
5'1"
5'0"
4'11"
4'10"
Pounds  50      75        100       125       150       175       200       225       250

* Without shoes
  Without clothes. The higher weights apply to people with more muscle and bone, such as many men.
  Source: Report of the Dietary Guidelines Advisory Committee on the Dietary Guidelines for Americans, 1995.

## Diabetes

Diabetes, or high blood sugar, is a serious disorder that raises the risk of coronary heart disease. The risk of death from heart disease is about three times higher in women with diabetes. Diabetic women also are more apt to have high blood pressure and high blood cholesterol.

Diabetes is often called a "woman's disease" because after age 45 about twice as many women as men develop diabetes. While there is no cure for this disorder, there are steps a person can take to control it. In certain people, being overweight and growing older are linked with the development of the most common type of diabetes. Losing excess weight and boosting physical activity may help postpone or prevent the disease.

## Other Factors

### Stress

In recent years, we have heard a lot about the connection between stress and heart disease. For example, studies have found that the most commonly reported incident preceding a heart attack is an emotionally upsetting event, particularly one that involves anger. Also, some common ways of coping with stress, such as over-eating, heavy drinking, and smoking, are clearly bad for your heart.

The good news is that sensible health habits can have a protective effect. Regular physical activity not only relieves stress, but can directly lower your risk of heart disease. Also, participating in a stress management program following a heart attack lowers the chances of further heart-related problems.

Studies also suggest that having emotionally supportive relationships lessens the chances of developing heart disease and prolongs life following a heart attack. While these findings are promising, researchers will need to conduct further studies to find out more about the links among certain behaviors, stress, and coronary heart disease in women.

## Birth Control Pills

Birth control pills (oral contraceptives) used to have much higher doses of estrogen than they do today. Such pills increased the risk of vascular and heart disease, especially among women who smoked.

Today, "high-dose" refers to pills containing about 50 micrograms of estrogen. However, American women much more commonly use "low-dose" pills that have 35 micrograms of estrogen or less. There is little, if any, additional risk of heart disease for premenopausal women using a pill that has up to 50 micrograms of estrogen.

However, taking a birth control pill does pose risks for some women. If you are now taking any kind of birth control pill or are considering using one, keep these guidelines in mind:

- If you smoke cigarettes, stop smoking or consider a different form of birth control. Smoking boosts the risks of serious cardiovascular problems from birth control pill use, especially the risk of blood clots, and particularly in women over 35.

- Use of birth control pills may increase blood pressure. If you take oral contraceptives, you should get your blood pressure checked regularly. If you develop hypertension, you should ask your doctor about changing pills or switching to another form of birth control.

- If you take birth control pills and are diabetic or prediabetic, you should have regular blood sugar tests.

- If you have had problems with blood clots, a heart attack, or a stroke, or if you have any other kind of cardiovascular disease, oral contraceptives may not be a safe choice. Be sure your doctor knows about your condition before prescribing birth control pills for you.

Of course, this addresses only cardiovascular points. For a more complete discussion about birth control pills, talk with your doctor.

## Homocysteine

Homocysteine (pronounced homo-SIS-teen) is an amino acid that is found normally in the body. Recent studies suggest that high blood levels of this substance may increase a person's chances of developing heart disease, stroke, and reduced blood flow to the hands and feet. It is believed that high levels of homocysteine may damage the arteries, make the blood more likely to clot, and/or make blood vessels less flexible.

Recent research also shows that the level of homocysteine in the blood is affected by the consumption of three vitamins—folic acid and vitamins B6 and B12. People who consume less than the recommended daily amounts of these vitamins are more likely to have higher homocysteine levels. Recommended daily amounts are as follows: 400 micrograms of folic acid, 2 milligrams of B6, and 6 micrograms of B12.

It has not yet been proven that lowering homocysteine levels will actually help to prevent heart or blood vessel disease. But, until

---

*People who drink heavily on a regular basis have higher rates of heart disease than either moderate drinkers or nondrinkers.*

---

more research is done, women can help protect their health by getting enough folic acid, B6, and B12 in their diets.

Good sources of folic acid include citrus fruits, tomatoes, vegetables, whole-grain and fortified-grain products, beans, and lentils. Foods high in B6 include meat, poultry, fish, fruits, vegetables, and grain products. Major sources of B12 are meat, poultry, fish, and milk and other dairy products.

## Alcohol

Several recent studies have reported that moderate drinkers—those who have one or two drinks per day—are less likely to develop heart disease than people who don't drink any alcohol. If you are a nondrinker, this is not a recommendation to start using alcohol. And certainly, if you are pregnant or have another health condition that could make alcohol use harmful, you should not drink. But if you are already a moderate drinker, you may be less likely to have a heart attack.

But remember, moderation is the key. More than three drinks per day can raise blood pressure, and binge drinking can lead to stroke. People who drink heavily on a regular basis have higher rates of heart disease than either moderate drinkers or nondrinkers.

The "Dietary Guidelines for Americans" recommend that for overall health, women should have no more than one drink per day. One drink equals 12 ounces of beer, or 5 ounces of wine, or 1 1/2 ounces of 80-proof liquor.

Keep in mind, too, that alcohol provides no nutrients—only extra calories. If you are trying to control your weight, you may want to cut down on alcohol and substitute calorie-free iced tea, mineral water, or seltzer.

## Hormones and Menopause

Should menopausal women use hormone pills? There is no simple answer to this question.

Menopause is caused by a decrease in estrogen produced by a woman's ovaries. As estrogen levels begin to drop, some women develop uncomfortable symptoms such as "hot flashes" and mood changes. Hormone replacement therapy (HRT)—a term for prescription hormone medications—can be used to relieve these symptoms. Some women are prescribed medication that contains only estrogen. Others take estrogen combined with a second hormone, called progestin.

### *Hormone Therapy and Heart Health*

The latest research indicates that HRT may have important heart benefits for women after menopause. The National Institutes of Health (NIH) supported a major study on HRT called the Postmenopausal Estrogen/Progestin Interventions (PEPI) Trial. It found that HRT raised levels of HDL and decreased those of LDL. This was true for both HRT with estrogen alone or in combination with progestin.

Further, HRT slowed the bone loss that occurs with menopause and significantly increased bone mass. These effects on bone were strongest among older women and those who had not recently used hormones. Smokers, who generally lose bone mass more quickly than nonsmokers, gained as much bone on average as nonsmokers.

HRT did not increase blood pressure or cause weight gain.

There was a key difference between the estrogen-only and estrogen-progestin forms of HRT and their effects on the uterine lining, called the endometrium. HRT using estrogen plus progestin prevented overgrowth of the uterine lining, while HRT with estrogen-only increased the risk of such overgrowth.

### *Deciding on HRT*

Some questions about HRT remain. For example, PEPI was not large enough and did not last long enough to examine breast cancer issues. However, other research suggests HRT slightly increases that risk, perhaps only in women who take it for 5 or more years.

To decide whether or not to use HRT, talk with your doctor or health professional about your risk of heart disease, osteoporosis (a severe thinning of the bones that makes them more likely to break), cancer, your family medical history, and quality of life issues.

In addition, these guidelines may help in deciding on HRT:

- Postmenopausal women who have not had a hysterectomy (removal of the uterus) should consider taking a therapy that combines estrogen with progestin or natural progesterone. A woman with a uterus who decides to take estrogen-only should have a yearly endometrial biopsy (an examination of the uterine lining).

- Postmenopausal women who have had a hysterectomy would get no additional cardiovascular or bone-mass benefit from adding a progestin. They are not at risk for overgrowth of the uterine lining.

Finally, if you decide to use HRT, you should periodically review your status with your health professional. And be alert for signs of trouble, especially abnormal bleeding, dizziness, or severe headaches, and immediately report these to the doctor. They may or may not be due to the HRT.

## Aspirin

The research on aspirin is promising: This well-known "wonder drug" may help to both prevent and treat heart attacks. A study of more than 87,000 women found that those who took a low dose of aspirin regularly were less likely to suffer a first heart attack than women who took no aspirin. Women over age 50 appeared to benefit most.

Other recent research suggests that only a tiny daily dose of aspirin may be needed to protect against heart attacks. One study found that, for both women and men, taking only 30 mg of aspirin daily—one-tenth the strength of a regular aspirin—helped prevent heart attacks as effectively as the usual 300 mg dose. The smaller dose also caused less stomach irritation.

Aspirin also reduces the chances that women who have already had a heart attack or stroke will have, or die from, another one. If taken quickly, aspirin may also increase the chances of survival after a heart attack.

Keep in mind, however, that aspirin is a powerful drug with many side effects. It can increase your chances of getting ulcers, kidney disease, liver disease, and a stroke from a hemorrhage. Because of these serious risks, you should not take aspirin to either prevent or treat a heart attack without first discussing it with your doctor.

# The Quiet Enemy[3]

By MARCIA MATTSON
*FLORIDA TIMES-UNION,* OCTOBER 2, 2001

In an era when deaths from several cancers are declining, ovarian cancer has emerged as the most deadly form of gynecologic cancer.

The cancer is difficult to detect and diagnose. It can develop quietly, without causing any outwardly apparent symptoms. When symptoms do develop, they tend to be so mild and general that women and many doctors mistake them for signs of other ailments.

That has led some doctors to call ovarian cancer "the whispering disease." Ovarian cancer first whispered, then shouted, its presence to Carolyn Webb of Jacksonville as she traveled from internist to gynecologist to gastroenterologist over nearly two years, looking for answers to why she had become plagued with indigestion and bloating. She started to thicken in her abdomen. Her clothing had to be altered.

"I thought, oh well, I'm just spreading," Webb said.

Her gastroenterologist raised a concern about ovarian cancer because Webb had entered her 50s and was going through menopause, the time when most ovarian cancers develop.

But an ultrasound and a CT scan, she was told, didn't detect any sign of cancer.

"Then that just sort of was off our list," she said. "I never thought of it again."

Doctors checked the health of her colon, stomach and gall bladder. And Webb developed additional and more painful symptoms, including constipation, frequent urination and lower back pain.

By the time she received another CT scan in 1999, cancerous tumors blanketed one area of her abdomen. Her husband, Warner, a pediatrician, saw the CT scan result first.

"When I saw his face, I knew I was in big trouble," Webb said.

The trouble doctors had in diagnosing Webb is commonplace. Seventy-five percent of ovarian cancers still are diagnosed in the late stages, when they are difficult to treat and the likelihood of death is greater. Ovarian cancer death rates haven't dropped much in 40 years.

One in every 65 American women get the disease. More than 23,000 women will be diagnosed this year, and about 13,900 will die—mainly because they won't be diagnosed with the cancer until it has grown too difficult to treat.

"Everybody we know that had the disease had the same story," her husband said.

She was diagnosed with late-stage ovarian cancer. The tumors produced fluid that were causing many of her symptoms.

Webb underwent a six-hour surgery to remove her ovaries, two parts of her colon, a tumor from her liver, some lymph nodes and part of her stomach. Her uterus had been removed years ago, or it would have been part of the surgery as well. Bernd-Uwe Sevin, chairman of Mayo Clinic Jacksonville's department of obstetrics and gynecology, performed the surgery with help from general surgeons and a liver specialist.

A cancerous ovary can expand to the size of a grapefruit without causing too much pain because the abdominal cavity is so spacious. But Webb's ovary hadn't expanded much. Instead, cancer cells had spread from it to other tissues.

Sevin said it's difficult to remove all of the tumors from abdominal tissue, so the goal is to reduce them, then use chemotherapy drugs that work well in killing the remaining cancer cells that scatter on abdominal surfaces "like snow in the forest—on all the branches, everywhere."

Doctors removed some of her bone marrow, in case she will need a transplant later. Then Webb underwent seven rounds of chemotherapy. Her granddaughter, Caroline, would lie down with her to take naps. And when most of Webb's hair fell out, the child gave her grandmother a play wig from her Little Mermaid costume.

"That's one of the things I cried the most about, to think I wasn't going to be here to do things with her," Webb said.

She also entered a clinical trial that dispersed mouse antibodies containing a radioactive substance throughout her abdomen. The goal is for the antibodies to attach to the surface of the cancer cells, and for the radiation to kill cells within a small radius. The process weakened Webb considerably, and her family supplied her with about 15 blood transfusions.

Today doctors can't find any sign of cancer.

"We're very thankful they were aggressive as they were," Webb said of her treatment physicians.

---

## Symptoms

Ovarian cancer usually causes no symptoms in its early stages, but in later stages may cause:

—Bloating.
—Indigestion.
—Changes in bowel habits.
—Pelvic pressure.
—Gas.
—Stomach pain.
—Back pain.
—Vaginal bleeding.
—Leg pain.

Women who are noticing these symptoms should talk to their doctor.

More women would be diagnosed earlier in their ovarian cancer if patients and physicians took a few basic steps, Sevin said.

The first step is an annual gynecologic exam that includes both a manual vaginal exam and a manual rectal exam, so the doctor can feel the ovaries' size and shape from two angles—from in front of the uterus and from behind it. This may help detect if an ovary is growing.

Too many doctors are not performing the manual rectal exam, Sevin said. Some doctors also are not asking their patients questions that would indicate the ovaries' health.

Doctors routinely ask if women feel abdominal pain, discomfort or burning. Those questions address problems with the uterus, Sevin said. Doctors should also ask patients if they have any symptoms linked with ovarian cancer, he said. A woman may not think to tell her gynecologist she is having bloating, gas or constipation because she may not think those symptoms have anything to do with her reproductive system. So the doctor must ask specific questions, Sevin said.

*Ovarian cancer, despite its deadliness, remains a relatively rare cancer, making up just 4 percent of all cases in women.*

Beyond a thorough annual exam, patients and doctors can pay more attention to risk factors for ovarian cancer, such as family histories of breast, colon or ovarian cancer. Researchers just recently developed better methods for predicting who is at higher risk, he said. Still, only 10 percent of ovarian cancers are thought to be hereditary. Women who never had children or had them late in life are also at increased risk.

There is no reliable screening test for ovarian cancer, as there is for prostate cancer, but a couple of diagnostic tools can help doctors with their detective work.

One is a blood test called the CA 125. This test is a marker for several kinds of cancer as well as a list of other ailments. It is a starting point if a woman's exam, symptoms and family history raise the possibility of ovarian cancer.

Also, the transvaginal ultrasound, performed by placing a scope-like device inside the pelvis, gives doctors a better view of the ovaries and surrounding tissue than the standard ultrasound, in which a device is placed over the woman's abdomen. Webb's initial ultrasound was a standard one. Sevin said it's important that the procedure be performed by someone who is skilled at interpreting the results.

Ovarian cancer, despite its deadliness, remains a relatively rare cancer, making up just 4 percent of all cases in women. So using these screening tests routinely on every woman wouldn't make economic sense or result in the finding of many more cases early, Sevin said.

# A Woman's Greatest Fear[4]

BY DONALD D. HENSRUD
*FORTUNE*, APRIL 15, 2002

Coronary heart disease kills almost six times more women than breast cancer does. Even so, if you ask a woman what disease she's most afraid of, her answer will likely be breast cancer.

There are many risk factors—obesity, having children late in life, hormone replacement therapy, beginning menstruation early and menopause late, the high-dose oral contraceptives that were popular years ago. The risk doubles if one first-degree relative has had breast cancer; it increases fivefold if more than one has been affected.

Only 5% to 10% of breast cancers are primarily due to genetic mutations, but the consequences are significant. For women with a strong family history of breast cancer, we'll check for two specific genes, BRCA1 and BRCA2. When a mutation has occurred, a prophylactic bilateral mastectomy can reduce the risk of developing breast cancer by more than 90%. Because of the horrifying implications for the patient and her daughters, our genetics counselors review and discuss the entire subject with the patient before genetic testing is performed.

For women who are at high risk, one preventive option is tamoxifen, a drug that decreases risk but can cause hot flashes, blood clots, and other side effects. Another drug being studied is raloxifene.

But what is frustrating is that some 75% of all breast cancers occur in women who are not obviously at risk. Although no one has demonstrated that self-exams improve outcome, the truth is that women, not their physicians, discover most lumps. We recommend checking once a month on the same date or just after the menstrual period, when fluid retention is least. If a new lump (they're usually painless) doesn't go away after one cycle, it's time to see a physician.

A recent study published in Britain's Lancet claimed that mammograms don't save lives by detecting breast cancer. Every medical institution has since had its say. Along with the Secretary of Health and Human Services and the American Cancer Society, Mayo firmly believes in yearly mammograms for women over 40.

---

4. Article by Donald D. Hensrud from *Fortune* April 15, 2002. Copyright © 2002 Time Inc. All rights reserved.

---

# Breast Cancer Myths

BY DIANE KOZAK
*PREVENTION*, AUGUST 15, 2001

Would turning off your electric blanket, switching to deodorant instead of antiperspirant, and going braless really cut your risk of breast cancer? Since researchers haven't fully solved the puzzle of why women get breast cancer, many of us—experts and regular folks alike—have theorized about possible links to everyday activities, says Robert A. Smith, PhD, director of cancer screening for the American Cancer Society in Atlanta.

**Here's the truth:** While extensive research shows that breast cancer has many causes—hormonal, environmental, genetic, and dietary—don't worry about these false alarms:

## Electric Blankets

**Theory:** Harvard University researchers speculated that exposure to low-level electromagnetic fields from electric blankets might raise risk by suppressing secretion of melatonin, a hormone that may be protective. **Reality:** The Nurse's Health Study of 87,497 women found no link (*Amer. Jour. of Epidemiology*, July 2000).

## Antiperspirants

**Myth:** An e-mail message widely circulated on the Internet fueled a persistent—and erroneous—rumor that antiperspirants prevented the release of toxins in underarm sweat. The toxins were said to get into lymph nodes and cause cancer. **Reality:** Wrong! While sweat does contain water, urea, and salt, it does not contain toxins. Second, sweat glands aren't connected to the lymph nodes.

## Bras

**Myth:** Bras constrict lymphatic tissue, allowing cancer-causing toxins to build up. **Reality:** "When I first heard this one, I thought, 'Surely you jest,'" Dr. Smith says. Bras—even tight-fitting ones—don't interfere with lymphatic drainage at all.

*Source:* Article by Diane Kozak from *Prevention* November 1998. Copyright © *Prevention*. Reprinted with permission.

---

If anything suspicious turns up on the first view, our radiologists pursue further evaluation with magnification views or ultrasound. If it's called for, we do a fine-needle or core biopsy, sometimes stereotactically (a 3-D process that pinpoints the area). If an open biopsy is required, a surgeon will step in.

Years ago the breast, the lymph nodes, and part of the underlying muscle were removed in most cases. We're much more conservative now. For small cancers, a lumpectomy followed by six weeks of radiation may be all that's needed. In many new cases, we'll sample at least one underarm lymph node as a guide to treatment. For large cancers or cancers that have spread, chemotherapy is an option.

Research is ongoing, and improvements are likely in the coming years. In the meantime, the debate over mammography has, if nothing else, alerted the world to the huge number of breast-cancer survivors. In fact, when breast cancer is detected and treated at an early stage, a woman has a greater than 95% chance of still being alive five years later.

# "Why Don't They Just Eat?"[5]

BY JENNIFER PIRTLE
*HEALTH*, MARCH 2002

Unlike many women who develop an eating disorder, Shannon Hurd did not grow up preoccupied with food. As a 16-year-old, she'd lunch on a cheeseburger and fries while her fellow high school cheerleaders picked over their minuscule salads. But when the young man whom Hurd, now 24, remembers as her first love, abruptly ended their relationship, everything changed for her. She soon plummeted into a deep depression and became anorexic. Over the course of the next several months, Hurd lost more than 50 pounds from her athletic 6-foot frame, dropping from 165 to 113.

Yet despite her ghostly pallor and the tendons that protruded, rope-like, through her skin, it wasn't until Hurd suffered a heart attack in 1994 that she realized, with horrifying clarity, the degree to which her eating habits had ravaged her body. Although she has now made it back to 165 and kept her weight stable there for nearly five years, Hurd still gingerly navigates the road to psychological well-being. Currently a graduate student at the University of Colorado at Boulder, she says she has developed a lifesaving—but rigid—eating plan. She has dumped boyfriends and quit jobs just to avoid missing breakfast or lunch, nutritional lapses she fears might unravel the progress she's made. "Maintaining my weight is a full-time job," she says. "I didn't understand how complex recovery would be."

One reason women like Hurd have such difficulty overcoming eating disorders is that experts have never been able to nail down a specific cause, Of course, many people blame social pressures—the media's obsession with stick-thin models, for instance, or a mother's overbearing control of her daughter's diet. But biology, not society, may be the root of eating disorders. Some groundbreaking new research suggests that such factors as brain chemistry and genetics may set a woman up to develop a disorder later in life. This research could lay the groundwork for more effective treatments for eating disorders, including drug and gene therapy. Better yet, it might allow doctors to predict who is predisposed to developing them, allowing those women to get treatment before suffering emotionally and physically damaging illnesses.

---

That's big news because, according to conservative estimates, eating disorders affect between 5 million and 10 million young women in the United States. This year, at least 50,000 individuals will die as a direct result of an eating disorder. "Currently, these disorders have the highest rates of death of any psychiatric illness, but we have not understood why women get them," says Walter Kaye, M.D., professor of psychiatry at the University of Pittsburgh Medical Center. "If we can identify a population that is at risk, we are more likely to be successful in preventing the disorders."

Kaye is spearheading an international research project on the genetics of women with anorexia and bulimia. He first became interested in tracking the biology of these illnesses when he noticed particular patterns in eating-disorder patients: The disorders occur mainly in women, they begin at an early age, they seem to run in families, and they produce similar symptoms in patients. "To my mind, this suggests that there is some biological contributing factor," Kaye says.

Under Kaye's leadership, teams of researchers have been working with about 4,000 female participants for the past five years at centers in Germany, Italy, Canada, and five locations throughout the United States to unlock both the biological and genetic causes of eating disorders. Studies at the University of Pittsburgh are using brain-imaging scans to help identify regions of the brain that may make people more susceptible to developing eating disorders, particularly those regions that are affected by the serotonin system. The brain compound serotonin, derived from tryptophan—an amino acid found only in food—is involved in the transmission of nerve impulses, and helps regulate mood, impulse control, and appetite levels. When people eat, their serotonin levels rise, contributing to satiety.

*In women with anorexia, some component of the serotonin system seems to be out of whack.*

But in women with anorexia, some component of the serotonin system seems to be out of whack. Hurd and other women who have had eating disorders often speak of the calmness and the intense pleasure that comes from not eating. "Anorexics would not do this unless it felt good," she says. Bulimics, as well, often report feelings of satisfaction after binge eating and purging.

To try to understand the pattern, Kaye's researchers compared levels of serotonin in women who were recovered from anorexia or bulimia for at least a year with healthy volunteers who had never had an eating disorder. They found that young women who have suffered from eating disorders have unusually high levels of serotonin. Researchers don't yet know if these differences in serotonin levels are the cause of anorexia and bulimia—or the result—but this discovery might be able to explain why women with eating disorders feel full even when they haven't had food for days.

Kaye's research into some genetic component to eating disorders is highly preliminary, but it is just as provocative as the serotonin studies. At Kaye's study site at the University of California at Los Angeles, researchers discovered that women who had a family history of anorexia nervosa were 12 times more likely to develop the disorder. Women with bulimia in their families were four times more likely to become bulimic themselves. And studies done at Kaye's other collaborative sites—including the Neuropsychiatric Research Institute in North Dakota and sites in Virginia, Minnesota, and Australia—have shown similar results, both within families and in studies of twins.

These studies are merely the first steps toward isolating the specific genes that cause eating disorders. Kaye and his researchers say that may not happen for years, in part because they suspect many genes play a role. "In addition to the numerous genes, there are many cultural and psychosocial issues that are involved too, which makes isolating the direct causes difficult," explains James Mitch-

---

*"If we could further narrow the age range of women who are susceptible to eating disorders, for instance, that would be very important."*—Suzanne Johnson, Adult Weight and Eating Disorders Program (Boston)

---

ell, M.D., president of the Neuropsychiatric Research Institute and one of Kaye's colleagues.

Kaye and his team of scientists are hopeful that their work will eventually lead to more successful treatments. Targeted medications could revolutionize the recovery from eating disorders, much as they have helped people with clinical depression, a disorder that also has a brain-chemistry component. And Mitchell says that with some recent advances in genetics research, gene therapy could be a possibility sometime in the future. "Some things that appear to be genetically preordained can be modified," he says.

But still, the most promising implications are in the area of prevention. Once the genetic research is complete, it is possible that doctors could be able to identify high-risk women by their genotypes and to offer preventive treatment before their disorders surface. Suzanne Johnson, Ph.D., a psychologist in the Adult Weight and Eating Disorders Program at Massachusetts General Hospital in Boston, says that the potential impact of this kind of prevention is tremendous. "Kaye's work could certainly be very helpful on a predictive level," she says. "If we could further narrow the age range of women who are susceptible to eating disorders, for instance, that would be very important."

Johnson also believes the research into the genetic and biological causes of eating disorders might help therapists who are working with eating-disorder patients. "Women with eating disorders are dealing with so much shame," Johnson says. "If we had a biological or genetic basis for these disorders, it may help them understand why they are predisposed to this set of symptoms, and may help alleviate that shame."

As for Shannon Hurd, she hopes that at the very least, this new research might change public perception of the illness and silence the whispered refrain of "Why don't they just eat?" After all, Hurd says, overcoming her anorexia wasn't simply about putting fork to food. "It's definitely not a disease about dieting," she says. "I never wanted to ruin my life."

# The Menopause Decision

## True Stories from Real Women[6]

By Dahpna Caperonis
*Natural Health*, April 2002

All women face a crossroads at menopause: whether or not replenish lost estrogen and other sex hormones. Some women want proven relief from frustrating problems like hot flashes. Others hope to prevent heart disease, osteoporosis, or other signs of aging linked to low hormone levels. Against these positives, any woman must weigh the downsides of hormone replacement therapy (HRT), like weight gain and possible breast cancer risk.

Compounding matters, there are now dozens of natural and synthetic HRT options. How do you choose? Prioritize, says Stephen Sinatra, M.D., the author of *Heart Sense for Women* (Plume, 2001) and a cardiologist in Manchester, Conn., who has treated hundreds of women approaching menopause. First, consider how menopause-related problems like hot flashes have affected your quality of life. Then find out if you are at increased risk for estrogen-related ailments like osteoporosis and heart disease. And during this process, of course, work with your health care practitioner to find the best therapy for you.

Two women, Susan Graham and Joan Alix, could hardly have predicted the journey they'd take as they faced the crossroads of menopause. Each tried several forms of hormone replacement therapy before finding their direction. Their stories illustrate how to choose your path and make the right HRT decision.

### Susan Graham

Susan Graham was a straight-A student in high school and college, and in graduate school she easily grasped the complexities of neurology. So the Manchester, Conn.-based licensed practical nurse was more than surprised when, in her mid-30s, she couldn't remember the magazine paragraph she had just read.

As Graham was losing her powers of concentration, intense hot flashes began to overwhelm her. "I felt like I had a chronic sunburn," she says. "[The surges] stopped me in my tracks. I was absolutely drenched." The hot flashes came daily, slowly at first and by evening, every 10 minutes. She also became severely depressed.

---

6. Copyright © April 2002, *Natural Health*, Weider Publications, Inc. Reprinted with permission.

When she passed tests for everything from blood cell counts to heart irregularities, Graham was puzzled. In some ways, being a health care professional made it easier for her to handle the constant evaluations and to talk to her doctors. But it also made the lack of answers harder to bear. Besides hot flashes and the bizarre brain fog, Graham had unusually heavy periods. All three are signs that the ovaries have stopped producing regular levels of hormones, so Graham asked her gynecologist if she could be approaching menopause. Her gynecologist said no. (Typically, symptoms don't begin until a woman is 39 to 45 years old.)

*Women can lose up to 20 percent of bone mass in the five to seven years after menopause.*

Three gynecologists and 18 months later, Graham remembers begging a doctor, "Please humor me and test me for menopause." Finally, at age 39, she got a positive diagnosis.

### The Search for Relief

Menopause before age 40, or premature menopause, happens to about 8 percent of women. Graham's doctors immediately checked for known (but rare) causes of premature menopause like brain tumors and lupus. Those tests came up negative. "The most likely explanation is that I simply ran out of eggs," says Graham.

Graham read every book she could find on menopause, which 10 years ago was only a handful of titles. The most comprehensive one touted estrogen replacement. But Graham knew that reports dating from the mid-'70s had associated estrogen with an increased risk of breast cancer. "No women in her right mind takes [that risk] lightly," she says.

Graham decided to try alternative medicine first because of her interest in natural remedies. "I don't like to start prescription medication unless it's necessary," explains Graham. "I figure, if I can handle a problem with a BB gun, why bring out a cannon?" She tried soy and the herbs dong quai (Angelica sinensis), black cohosh (Cimicifuga racemosa), and red clover (Trifolium pratense), as well as acupressure, massage, and yoga.

Unfortunately, even after a few months, nothing worked, she says, "not even one bit."

### On to Plan B

Graham decided to try conventional medicine. By then, it wasn't a difficult decision. "I was miserable. My whole being was unraveling—mentally, emotionally, and physically," she says. "My body was screaming for estrogen." Graham also knew that the longer she lacked estrogen, the more vulnerable her small frame would be

---

# The Hormone Options Explained

Get to know your treatment options so you can ask your doctor specific questions. Here are seven common versions of hormone replacement therapy (HRT).

1. ESTROGENS (NATURAL)—Called natural because they mimic the hormones in your body, these estrogens are synthesized from plants or animals. There are three natural estrogens: estrone, estriol, and estradiol.

2. ESTROGENS (CONJUGATED)—A mixture of several forms of estrogen (some of them are natural to animals, but not humans). Premarin, the most widely prescribed of this type, comes from pregnant mares' urine.

3. ESTROGENS (COMPOUNDED)—Prescription combinations of natural estrogens. They are prepared by special compounding pharmacies and are available as "biest" (estrone and estradiol) or "triest" (estrone, estradiol, and estriol).

4. PROGESTERONE (CREAM)—A topical treatment synthesized in a lab from plants such as wild yam (Discorea composita). It is considered natural because it is structurally identical to the progesterone in your body. Note: Wild yam cream does not contain progesterone.

5. PROGESTERONE (MICRONIZED)—A natural progesterone made up of tiny coated particles that prevent your stomach from destroying the hormones. It appears to have fewer side effects than synthetic progesterone.

6. PROGESTERONE (SYNTHETIC)—Form of the hormone that differs chemically from what your body produces. Sometimes known as progestin, it may be derived from natural sources. Provera is the most common synthetic form.

7. TESTOSTERONE—The main sex hormone in men is also produced in women's ovaries and dwindles after menopause. Supplemental testosterone may increase libido. Available in synthetic pill form and as a natural cream or gel.

---

to osteoporosis. Women can lose up to 20 percent of bone mass in the five to seven years after menopause; at 39, Graham had the potential for living many years with brittle bones.

In 1991, she started Premarin, a combination of several estrogens called "conjugated estrogen." (For a glossary of HRT types, see "The Hormone Options Explained.") In a few days, she was sleeping all night and her hot flashes had disappeared. In about two weeks, her brain felt sharp again. She felt better than she had in years. But the bliss lasted only three weeks.

The problems began when Graham started taking Provera, a synthetic form of progesterone. (Progesterone reduces the high risk of uterine cancer that occurs with taking estrogen by itself.) Right away she developed headaches, body aches, bloating, exhaustion, and extreme irritability. Over several tortuous months, her doctor reduced her dose. Finally, with her doctor's permission, she tried micronized progesterone, a natural form that gave her fewer side effects.

One year ago, Graham switched from Premarin to estradiol, a prescription drug that's considered a natural estrogen because it has the same molecular structure as the estrogen made in a woman's body. Today, "I feel great," she says.

## Making Peace with Menopause

Coping with the change of life was especially hard for Graham, because she was so young. "There was no one to talk to about the infertility aspect," she says. "I felt barren. That was the hardest thing, psychologically." It took her years to work through the grieving process.

Graham has advice for women of any age: "Read everything you can get your hands on," she recommends. "The more you know, the more powerful you are." It's also important to find a gynecologist you can work with and to get regular diagnostic testing (like bone scans, hormonal tests, and mammography). Finally, be open-minded. "I've seen women suffer for years trying to make natural therapies work," says Graham. "Don't beat yourself up if conventional medicine turns out to be the best option for you."

## Joan Alix

Four years ago, Joan Alix began waking up nights swimming in perspiration. "I'm a flannel nightgown person," she says, but the sweats were so intense that she had to sleep practically nude. They came more often, exhausting her. And her periods became heavier and less frequent.

The timing of these health changes could not have been worse: Alix, then 51, was worrying about a father ailing from congestive heart failure; building a new home in Quonochontaug, R.I. (where she now lives); and adjusting to a new position as an elementary and middle school assistant principal. She thought stress brought on the sweats. Oh no, said her gynecologist; Alix was simply nearing menopause and, at her age, she should be taking hormones. She handed Alix a pharmaceutical brochure and three months' worth of sample estrogen-and-testosterone pills.

The kind of person who rarely takes medicine, Alix wasn't about to treat hormone pills lightly, but her father's heart condition prompted her to consider them. (Some evidence suggests that HRT reduces heart disease risk.) So did her gynecologist's demeanor. "It is intimidating when the doctor says 'Take this,'" says Alix.

Conflicted, she pored over books and articles about menopause. The more she read and thought, the more she realized that one prescription simply couldn't be right for everybody. She threw out her doctor's samples and continued to suffer night sweats and irregular periods.

A month or two later, Alix read a book about natural progesterone cream, a treatment that appeared to relieve fatigue and heavy periods. She also learned about Remifemin, a standardized form of the herb black cohosh that has estrogenlike effects in the body. Armed with this information, Alix starting taking the two remedies without consulting her gynecologist.

### Troubling Changes, Again

Alix quickly sensed that something just wasn't right. She felt bloated, she gained nearly 15 pounds in six months, and for the first time in her life she started craving starchy and sugary foods. Her night sweats and irregular periods continued. Fed up with a body that seemed to belong to someone else, she phoned Stephen Sinatra, M.D., a Manchester, Conn.-based cardiologist whose private practice was a short drive from her home. Alix's father had been seeing Sinatra for heart disease, and Alix was impressed by her dad's improvement.

Although Sinatra agreed that progesterone cream was a good therapy for some women, Alix's bloating, weight gain, and cravings led him to suspect that she was applying too much. He first lowered her dose and then asked her to stop using the progesterone cream altogether, so he could monitor her true hormone levels. For this purpose, he also asked Alix to stop taking Remifemin. For reasons still unknown, Alix's night sweats then subsided, a year after they began.

To address her weight gain and remaining symptoms, Sinatra concluded that Alix should try nonhormonal supplements and lifestyle changes. As a bonus, they would also help her manage her heart disease risk, he said. He recommended that Alix take a daily multivitamin plus vitamin E, magnesium, coenzyme $Q_{10}$, l-carnitine, and omega-3 fatty acids. He also advised her to eat more flaxseeds and cold-water fish and to walk more.

As Alix began trying Sinatra's recommendations, she took stock of her situation. She knew that her image of herself (as a young 125-pound woman who could eat whatever she wanted) no longer matched her reality. She now had to contemplate every piece of food that she put in her mouth and had to face up to a tough fact—she was getting older.

### Gathering Her Support Team

Gradually Alix realized she wasn't alone in her struggles. She called three aunts who are in their 70s and early 80s. These women stayed healthy and slim the way that Alix's northern Italian grand-

# How to Know If HRT Is the Right Treatment

To feel your best after menopause, you may need hormone replacement therapy (HRT). Additionally, HRT can lower the risk of some diseases that become more prevalent after menopause. But not everyone should take hormones. We asked Stephen Sinatra, M.D., a Manchester, Conn.-based cardiologist who treats menopausal women, to recommend treatments for 10 typical scenarios. He advises all women to take a multivitamin and regularly do weight-bearing and aerobic exercise. Before you decide on a treatment plan, talk to your health care practitioner.

| IF YOUR HEALTH RISK IS . . . | AND MENOPAUSE BRINGS ON . . . No Menopause Symptoms | AND MENOPAUSE BRINGS ON . . . Hot Flashes, Night Sweats, or Vaginal Dryness |
|---|---|---|
| No Risk | To slow aging and stay at no disease risk, try only lifestyle changes, including exercising and eating cold-water fish, flaxseeds, and soy, foods rich in healthy fats and protective plant estrogens. | Start with lifestyle changes (described at left). If you get no relief, try natural HRT (like estrogen cream and micronized progesterone). If ineffective, consider conjugated estrogens and synthetic progesterone. |
| Risk of Heart Disease | For 90 percent of cases, no HRT. If tests have shown high blood levels of fibrinogen and lipoprotien Lp(a), consider HRT if lifestyle changes cannot alter these factors. | Same as no risk (above). If tests have shown high blood levels of fibrinogen and lipoprotein Lp(a), consider HRT if lifestyle changes cannot alter these factors. |
| Risk of Breast Cancer | Try only lifestyle changes (avoid soy if you have had breast cancer). | Try only lifestyle changes (avoid soy if you have had breast cancer). |
| Risk of Osteoporosis | Try only lifestyle changes (consider HRT only if you have poor bone density). Also, get 10 to 15 minutes of sun exposure daily and take calcium and magnesium. | Same as no risk (top), and include sun exposure and minerals described at left. |
| Risk of Alzheimer's | Try only lifestyle changes. Also, take alpha lipoic acid, coenzyme $Q_{10}$, vitamin B complex, and vitamin E. | Same as no risk (top), and include the supplements described at left. |

parents did—by eating legumes like lentils, lean protein like fish, and plenty of fruits and vegetables, but little processed food. Alix decided to adopt this European way of eating. In a year, Alix lost the extra weight, evened out her cravings, and boosted her energy.

Alix visited her mother, 77, more often and found strength in her optimism and faith. She also looked to her church for support. A spiritual seminar it held, called "Life and the Spirit," was a watershed event for Alix. As her fellow parishioners shared stories of personal milestones, Alix began to reflect on who she was and what she wanted. The experience was reinforced by a favorite book, *The Wisdom of Menopause* (Bantam, 2001) by Yarmouth, Maine-based gynecologist Christiane Northrup, M.D. Northrup emphasizes that menopause is an important time in life to stop and regroup. "I look back at those years, and I think of Dr. Sinatra, my parents, husband, and two sons, and my faith, and those good influences are connected in my mind," says Alix.

Investigative reading and keeping in touch with her general practitioner and Sinatra remain Alix's top menopause strategies. "Women's bodies don't stop changing when they're 55," she says. "So you have to keep paying attention." Since the events of September 11, Alix has continued to connect with others; she prays regularly with friends and family. "Today more than ever, I'm making a conscious personal effort to be thankful," she says.

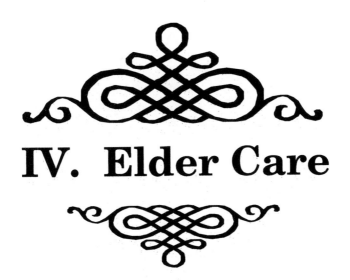

# IV. Elder Care

# Editor's Introduction

Geriatric medicine, caring for the elderly, and the role of Medicare in the lives of those over 65 are issues that are soon to be at the top of many Americans' priority list as the baby-boomer generation approaches retirement. Few people realize what sort of political, economic, and social impact this large demographic group is going to have on the country in just a few years. While those who belong to this aging generation need to plan for their own future financial and medical needs, their children will probably have to arrange for their care when they can no longer care for themselves. In addition, younger people are contributing their tax dollars toward government programs supporting their elders, whose number surpasses those who will contribute to the next generation's retirement funds, thus creating a shortage of money for this younger group when they retire. Health care for the elderly is therefore an issue that concerns all Americans. This chapter looks at the most pressing health care dilemmas facing the elderly and those who care for them. Because such a large number of people will soon enter the ranks of the country's senior citizens, it is important for everyone to learn what kinds of medical attention this aging population will require.

One of the most frightening and mysterious diseases of old age is Alzheimer's disease (AD). Afflicting 10 percent of those 65 and older and 50 percent of those 85 and older, AD appears to be caused by protein plaques that develop in the brain and eventually destroy it. Although pharmaceutical companies are trying to create drugs that will prevent or arrest the illness, no cure has been found yet. Diane Y. Chapman and Dan Osterweil look at AD, its various stages, and the role fitness professionals can play in improving the quality of life for patients.

Whether for AD or some other kind of malady, millions of senior citizens are prescribed medications every year, sometimes in staggering quantities. Many of these medications are unnecessary, addictive, or deadly when combined with others. Dr. Sanjay Gupta addresses the overmedication of seniors by examining the attitudes of doctors who prescribe the medications and asking why so many elderly patients are prescribed drugs they should not take to begin with.

The next article explores how drug companies are looking towards the baby-boomer generation for their next big payoff. Irene Alleger discusses the pharmaceutical industry and how drugs are being developed to combat the signs of aging. Though most studies indicate that nutrition, diet, and exercise are the keys to staying healthy and achieving longevity, the pharmaceutical companies are offering chemical alternatives in the form of new "anti-aging" creams and drugs. In a society that dotes on youth, this could prove to be the next big "wave" in medical research—not to mention a way for the pharmaceutical companies to become very rich.

The article that follows, "Fountains of Youth" by Sharon Begely, explores the highly controversial issue of stem cell research, which could potentially treat specific diseases that are caused by the aging process, as well as many of the illnesses discussed in this book. As Begley explains, some see the use of fetal stem cells as morally wrong, while others view it as the answer to all of humankind's medical problems. From cloning to gene research to cell replacement, stem cell research is the subject of much medical, political, and social debate.

Those seniors who require more intensive medical care may find themselves placed by their children or other care givers into nursing homes. Unfortunately, large cuts in Medicare are proving detrimental to these facilities. In "Long-Term Blues," Pamela Sherrid reports on the economics of the nursing home industry, which is complicated by reports of poor care in many facilities. As Sherrid explains, unless nursing homes address serious allegations of neglect and misconduct, the government may not assist them in their financial recovery.

Two alternatives to nursing home care for the terminally ill are hospice care and palliative care. A hospice is a homey environment that focuses on easing the experience of dying for individuals and their families during the last 6 months of life. Palliative care, on the other hand, helps to create a smooth transition for dying patients moving between the hospital and hospice care or home care. The last article in this section, "Dying in Peace," a personal account of Wendy Murray Zoba's visit to a palliative care unit in a Birmingham, Alabama, hospital, discusses the differences between hospice and palliative care and how each can play a role in the final days, weeks, or months of a person's life.

# Working with Clients with Alzheimer's Disease[1]

By Diane Y. Chapman
*IDEA Health & Fitness Source*, June 2001

While advances in medicine have extended our average life
expectancy, many of the diseases associated with aging continue to
challenge the scientific community. Chief among these is Alzheimer's disease (AD), which primarily afflicts older adults. AD is the
fourth leading cause of death in the United States, now affecting at
least 4 million adults (Institute for Brain Aging 2001). Some
experts estimate that 20 million people suffer from AD throughout
the world (Nash 2000).

The fitness industry stands poised to address the needs of this
growing population in ways you may not have even imagined.
Indeed, opting to work with people with AD may prove to be one of
the most fulfilling business decisions you ever make. If you are a
personal trainer, club owner, physical therapist community activity director or group fitness instructor, you can make a real contri-
bution to those afflicted with AD by creating exercise programs
that enhance their quality of life. Doing so will also give you an
edge in servicing a growing niche than is ripe with professional
possibilities.

## Our Aging Population

To understand why cases of AD are multiplying, it is helpful to
assess the growth of the senior segment of our population. According to the Assisted Living Federation of America (ALFA), the need
for services for seniors will expand continuously through the year
2050 owing to the following demographic changes in the U.S. population:

- the "graying" of the population

- the increase in the number of "frail elderly," described as persons over the age of 85

- the growth and development of existing and new health care,
  wellness and medical systems focused on providing options for
  the elderly (Gold et al. 1998)

---

1. Reproduced with permission of IDEA Health & Fitness Association, (800) 999-IDEA or
(858) 535-8979, *www.IDEAfit.com.*

Based on data from the U.S. Bureau of the Census, ALFA projects that the segment of the population 85 and older will increase 33.2 percent between the years 2000 and 2010 (Gold et al. 1998). By 2050, the number of Americans considered "frail elderly" could reach a high of 31.1 million. Citing the 6.5 million people 65 and older who currently need assistance with every day living—a number that is expected to rise to at least 13 million by 2020—ALFA predicts that job opportunities abound for those who can fulfill the "personal needs" of this population. Serving the fitness needs of seniors with Alzheimer's falls into this realm.

## Just What Is Alzheimer's Disease?

AD is just one of many causes of dementia, defined as a neuropsychological syndrome consisting of impairment of short-term memory, along with impairment of one or more of the following:

- language
- reasoning, logic or judgment
- spatial perception
- ability to perform planned motor actions
- insight
- other cognitive abilities (American Psychiatric Association 2000)

AD in particular has been described as "a progressive, degenerative disease of the brain that results in impaired memory, thinking and behavior" (Pfizer Inc. & Eisai Inc. 1997).

The cause of the disease is unknown, but genetic factors appear to play a role. The disease seems to run in some families and is influenced by several specific gene abnormalities (Berkow 1997). As parts of the brain degenerate, cells are destroyed and those cells that remain become unresponsive to many of the chemicals that transmit signals in the brain (Berkow 1997).

The pathology of AD is marked by the presence of brain tissue abnormalities called neurofibrillary tangles and neuritic plaque (Shankel 1999). The abnormal tissue first appears in the hippocampus and entorhinal cortex regions of the brain, then in the cortices of the frontal, parietal and temporal lobes. The hippocampus is the center of the autonomic nervous system; it creates and sends messages to the parts of the body that are needed to complete a desired task. The entorhinal cortex sends messages back and forth between the hippocampus and other parts of the brain. The frontal lobes help control mood and goal setting; the parietal lobes receive and process information about arithmetic, reading and body movement/sensation; and the temporal lobes process information about hearing, memory and language.

# 10 Warning Signs of Alzheimer's Disease

PATIENT CARE, NOVEMBER 15, 2001

The early detection of Alzheimer's disease is important. To help you, the Alzheimer's Association lists common warning signs and symptoms. Anyone who has several of these symptoms should contact a doctor for a thorough examination.

**1. Memory loss that affects job skills**
Occasionally forgetting an assignment, deadline, or coworker's name is normal, but frequent forgetfulness or unexplainable confusion may signal that something is wrong.

**2. Difficulty performing familiar tasks**
Busy people get distracted from time to time. For example, you might leave food on the stove too long or forget to serve part of a meal. In contrast, people with Alzheimer's disease might prepare a meal and not only forget to serve it but also forget they made it.

**3. Problems with language**
Everyone has trouble finding the right word sometimes, but a person with Alzheimer's disease may forget simple words or substitute inappropriate words, making his or her sentences difficult to understand.

**4. Disorientation to time and place**
Momentarily forgetting the day of the week or what you need from the store is normal. People with Alzheimer's disease, however, can become lost on their own street—not knowing where they are, how they got there, or how to get back home.

**5. Poor judgment**
Choosing not to wear a sweater or coat on a chilly night is a common mistake. A person with Alzheimer's disease, however, may dress inappropriately in more noticeable ways, such as wearing a bathrobe to the store or several blouses on a hot day.

**6. Problems with abstract thinking**
Balancing a checkbook can be challenging for many people, but for someone with Alzheimer's disease, recognizing numbers or doing basic math may be impossible.

**7. Misplacing things**
Everyone misplaces a wallet or keys from time to time. A person with Alzheimer's disease, however, may put items in inappropriate places—such as an iron in the freezer or a wristwatch in the sugar bowl—and then not recall how they got there.

**8. Changes in mood or behavior**
Everyone has many different emotions. People with Alzheimer's disease tend to have more rapid mood swings and overreact to minor stress.

**9. Changes in personality**
Our personalities may change somewhat as we age. But a person with Alzheimer's disease can change dramatically, usually over a period of time. For example, someone who was generally easygoing may become angry, paranoid, or afraid.

**10. Loss of initiative**
It is normal to tire of housework, a job, or social activities, but most people eventually regain their interest. The person with Alzheimer's disease may remain bored and uninvolved in activities he or she normally enjoyed.

*Source*: Used with permission: *Patient Care* 2001, 35:21. Thomson Healthcare Medical Economics.

Another characteristic of AD is the lowered production of brain chemicals such as acetylcholine, norepinephrine, serotonin and somatostatin, all of which affect normal communication between nerve cells. In the past, the only way to definitively diagnose AD was through autopsy. Recently, physicians have begun using magnetic resonance imaging (MRI) to diagnose the disease and detect its progression.

## Stages of Alzheimer's Disease

Although Alzheimer's patients may demonstrate varying degrees of severity and rates of disease progression, cognitive function declines in all cases. The stages of the disease are well-defined, as follows (Pfizer Inc. & Eisai Inc. 1997):

Stage I: Mild Alzheimer's Disease. This early stage typically lasts approximately two to four years. During this time, people with AD

---

*The most significant result of this new awareness of AD is the proliferation of facilities that provide skilled care and community support systems.*

---

commonly lose or misplace items such as keys; often forget names; and repeat statements or actions. They also begin to have difficulty remembering well-traveled routes and may become disinterested in activities they once enjoyed.

Stage II: Moderate Alzheimer's Disease. This stage lasts about two to 10 years. Mental abilities decline, and disruptive behavior is not uncommon. People become increasingly confused, agitated, argumentative and restless. They may even hallucinate. Because people with AD now require 24-hour care, this is usually when families or caretakers seek facilities for assistance.

Stage III: Severe Alzheimer's Disease. This final stage can last from one to three years. By now AD sufferers need help with all facets of daily living. They may not understand language and may fail to recognize family members—or even themselves in the mirror. It is during this final stage that they become susceptible to malnutrition, infections, pneumonia and other life-threatening diseases.

These three stages are the categories used most often in the clinical setting to define AD's progression. However, other assessment tools are also used to grade the disease's severity in terms of loss of cognitive and physical functioning. The Global Deterioration Scale breaks down the disease into seven stages (Reisberg 1982). The Functional Assessment Staging Tool describes a total of 16 successive stages and substages that track functional decline (Reisberg 1982). And the Brief Cognition Rating Scale is used to measure and define losses in concentration, memory, orientation and self-care.

## Changing Perceptions about AD

Because the senior population is growing, so too is the incidence of AD. "The incidence [of AD] grows with age. In the 65 to 74 age group, the incidence of AD is approximately 10 percent; from age 74 to 85, it is about 24.7 percent; and after age 85 it rises dramatically to over 40 percent. As we live longer with improved quality of physical life, we are statistically at risk for the deterioration of our mental abilities," says Loren B. Shook, president of the Alzheimer's Association of Orange County, California. He also serves as president and chief executive officer of Silverado Senior Living, a San Juan Capistrano, California, based organization that creates assisted-living communities throughout the United States. Silverado is also the first organization of its kind to create a pilot exercise initiative for AD residents in an assisted-living environment. . . .

As more and more people are stricken with AD, perceptions about the disease are starting to change. According to Wendy Graca, RN, BSN, Silverado's corporate director of health services, "In a culture that values cognition and control, it's easy to see why AD patients were reclusively treated for most of the [20th] century. Then, in the 1980s and 1990s, as medical science improved our life span dramatically, it became clear that AD was something that must be addressed in our elderly population. In fact, former president Ronald Reagan's condition and his family's openness about it raised the level of public support and knowledge dramatically."

The most significant result of this new awareness of AD is the proliferation of facilities that provide skilled care and community support systems. These care systems are the portal through which fitness professionals can enter the picture. "We believe there are changes that need to take place in the care institutions for AD, and we want to be in the forefront," says Shook. "One of those changes is the initiation of regular exercise programs for the residents. This one effort alone can give the elderly with AD a sense of freedom again: freedom to ambulate, freedom to move with more ease during daily activities and freedom to eat normally."

## Facilities for Seniors with AD

Silverado Senior Living communities are an example of assisted-living facilities in which management is determined to create a new paradigm of daily care for persons with AD. "The first thing we do in taking care of seniors with Alzheimer's is refer to them as 'residents' as opposed to calling them 'patients,'" says Shook. "Our philosophy is one of providing dignity in daily living, structuring our care to resemble the energy and activities of a typical American household. We do provide a full spectrum of medical care each day, but it is carefully downplayed to minimize its visual presence.

We don't want our residents to feel like they are in a hospital. Instead of seeing medical paraphernalia throughout the facility, you are more likely to see small dogs and cats in living rooms with fire-places."

Assisted-living communities are just one of the types of facilities that provide care for AD patients in the United States. According to Shook, there are 28,000 licensed assisted-living centers across the country, housing a population of more than 600,000 elderly. Other facilities that care for seniors with AD include nursing homes, continuing-care retirement communities and independent retirement communities. In addition, much of the AD care in this country is provided by family members in private homes. Senior community centers and adult day care centers help support families who care for AD sufferers at home.

For fitness professionals seeking to provide programs for this population, these facilities and services are excellent sources of potential clients. ALFA categorizes the different care facilities into four types:

**Assisted-Living Communities.** Assisted-living facilities are residential centers that offer the elderly a combination of housing, specialty support services and comprehensive medical care. These facilities focus on providing personalized care for those who need help with daily living; the centers are also equipped to meet medical needs, both scheduled or unscheduled in nature. Residents usually require assistance with the regular activities of daily living, such as bathing and dressing. According to ALFA, more than 1 million Americans currently reside in some type of assisted-living community. The residents' average age is 83.

**Nursing Homes.** These facilities provide round-the-clock medical care for patients who rely on assistance for all facets of daily care, such as bathing, dressing and using the toilet. Oftentimes, the patients in these homes also require medical interventions, such as feeding tubes.

**Continuing-Care Retirement Communities (CCRCs).** These residential communities provide many levels of care and assistance, such as independent living, assisted living and nursing home care. CCRCs usually provide health care, meals and a number of support services.

**Independent Retirement Communities (Congregate Living).** Primarily designed for active seniors, these communities provide group social events, home maintenance services, meals and house keeping. They do not provide medical or personal care.

## Effective Communication and Cuing Tips

Fitness professionals working with clients with Alzheimer's disease might want to employ these practices, suggested by the staff at Silverado Senior Living:

• Make and maintain eye contact with clients as often as possible.

• Identify yourself every time you meet with your clients. For example, you could say, "Hi, Mr. Smith, I'm Diane, your exercise instructor. Today, we are going to take a walk together." Remember, each time you see your clients, act as though you are meeting them for the first time. In their minds, you are.

• Use simple concepts and short words. Introduce and teach only one concept at a time. Do not link ideas or directions.

• Give a visual demonstration of each exercise or activity movement. Demonstrate just one option for any movement, based on fitness and skill level. Showing variations will only increase confusion.

• Ask for permission to touch clients with guided maneuvering hand cues so you can help them perform movements.

• Continue to prompt and cue each step of a movement with guided touch.

• Use concrete rewards to motivate clients each time you meet with them. These rewards can be as simple as a dish of ice cream, a pretty picture or a bowl of grapes. But remember that clients will need to see the reward (or at least a picture of it) to understand what you are referring to.

• Sustain concentration through focused attention and communication. Attention spans are short in this population.

## The Role of Fitness Professionals

As facilities that cater to AD sufferers continue to proliferate, so will your opportunities as a fitness professional. "The potential for any kind of service that helps this segment of our elderly is so tremendous," says Stephen F. Winner, MS, vice president of operations for Silverado Senior Living and the company's new "chief of culture." "Badly needed services can be anything from 'morning out' programs to adult day care centers to organized exercise and activity centers to home health services. It's all good and it all counts."

Winner, who sits on the Board of San Diego's Alzheimer's Association, enthusiastically endorses the concept of exercise for people with AD, provided that activities are designed around the specific limitations of the condition. "I know firsthand that Alzheimer's patients are being cared for in every type of setting, from private homes to senior centers to nursing homes, board and-care homes, assisted-living homes, churches and respite care centers. Caregivers and patients alike would find the addition of fitness programs refreshing and invigorating."

## Special Medical Considerations

When designing programs for seniors with AD, you must take into account the physical conditions that are typically present in this population: congestive heart failure; hypertension; asthma, emphysema and bronchitis; diabetes; arthritis and osteoporosis; and Parkinson's disease (Gifford 1999). The elderly are also particularly vulnerable to acute conditions, such as pneumonia, urinary-tract infections, strokes and fall-related traumas (especially hip fractures). Other conditions you need to consider when devising an exercise program for seniors with AD include poor vision, poor hearing, incontinence, depression, skin conditions and digestive disorders.

Poor vision, arthritis and neurological problems result in poor mobility and an unsteady gait (Gifford 1999). An unsteady gait can lead to falls and injuries. But research has shown that seniors who practice balance activities can avert the devastating effects of a fall (Perkins-Carpenter 2001).

"A common institutional response to the problems falls create is to decrease resident activity," says Shook. "In many facilities, AD residents are restrained to keep them from ambulating. Our observations indicate that when AD residents are restrained, their bodies deteriorate more rapidly. We keep detailed records of any falls in our residences, and we take a proactive approach to increase our residents' overall fitness levels to minimize falls. We have now shown that with aerobic activities, flexibility training and strength training, we can give back mobility to residents. This has resulted in reduced negative behaviors, reduction of the need for psychiatric medications and fewer medical restraints. Most important, our residents get a sense of being more in control of their lives in simple ways."

## Choosing Appropriate Activities

What types of exercise are appropriate for people with AD once they have been prescreened for medical concerns and have obtained the necessary physician approvals? Most experts suggest you start with flexibility and balance training. You can begin with an overall stretching routine, including neck stretches, and introduce some simple balancing exercises.

Another key component of any workout for seniors should be resistance training. According to the Keiser Corporation's Institute on Aging, numerous research studies have found that simple resistance training (e.g., leg presses, leg extensions and triceps extensions) can increase strength in frail, elderly subjects, even if they also suffer from arthritis, osteoporosis, diabetes or heart disease (Keiser 1999). One such study concluded that strength training activities can help prevent falls and loss of functional independence in subjects as old as 98 years of age (Fiatarone et al. 1994). When devising a resistance training program for clients with AD, you should ensure that exercises are chosen in accordance with the guidelines established in the American College of Sports Medicine's 1997 publication *Exercise Management for Persons with Chronic Diseases and Disabilities.* . . .

[Diane Y. Chapman is a freelance writer who specializes in health and fitness topics. She is the principal of Words To Your Advantage, a writing and speaking service based in Aliso Viejo, California. She is an ACE-certified group fitness instructor. Her father, Blair K. Chapman, died of Alzheimer's disease in October 1998.]

## References

American Psychiatric Association. 2000. *DSM-IV-TR.* Washington, DC: American Psychiatric Association.

Berkow, R. (Ed.) 1997. *The Merck Manual of Medical Information.* New York: Simon & Schuster Inc.

Cortes, C. W., et al. 1995. Effects of 16 weeks of high intensity strength training on frail adults with chronic disease. *Medicine & Science in Sports & Exercise.*

Davis, A. 2001. Assisted living firm prospers by housing a frail population. *Wall Street Journal,* ccxxxvi (10), Al.

Fiatarone, M. A., et al. 1994. Exercise training and nutritional supplementation for physical frailty in very elderly people. *New England Journal of Medicine,* 330 (June 23), 1769-75.

Gavzer, B. 2000. How can we help? *Parade Magazine* (July 16), 4.

Gifford, P. J. 1999. Medical conditions that can be treated in assisted living. *NIC Review,* 7: 97-103.

Gold, D., et al. 1998. The need for assisted living. *The Assisted Living Industry: An Overview.* Fairfax, VA: Assisted Living Federation of America.

Hadden, C., & Sattler, T. 2001. Management matters: Helping seniors get moving. *Fitness Management,* 17 (2), 41-4.

Hale, C. 2000. My father lost and found. *Health* (October), 136.

Institute for Brain Aging. 2001. What is dementia? *www.uci.edu/aboutad.html*; retrieved March.

Kluge, M. A., & Savis, J. 2000. Using chronobiology to enhance exercise quality for older adults. *ACSM's Health and Fitness Journal,* 4 (6), 20-5.

Kumpel, J.J., & Ransom, J. W. 1999. Supply-demand analysis: A current snapshot and look into the future. *NIC Review,* VII, 81-90.

Lasky, W. F. 1998. The current and future trends in assisted living. *The Assisted Living Industry: An Overview.* Fairfax, VA: Assisted Living Federation of America.

Lucas, C., & Schiffman, S. 1999. The essence of enhancement: Increasing residents' health & quality of life while increasing revenue. *NIC Review,* 7:35–41.

Nash, M. 2000. The new science of Alzheimer's. *Time* (July 17), 51.

Osterweil, D., Brummel-Smith, K., & Beck, J. C. 2000. *Comprehensive Geriatric Assessment.* New York: McGraw-Hill.

Perkins-Carpenter, B. P. 2001 Balance & stretching programs for seniors. *Fitness Management,* 17 (2), 32-4.

Pfizer Inc. and Eisai Inc. 1997. *Managing Alzheimer's Disease.* Pfizer Inc. and Eisai Inc.

Reisberg, B. 1982. The Global Deterioration Scale for the assessment of primary degenerative dementia. *American Journal of Psychiatry* 139:1136–39.

Shankel, W. R. 1999. Dr. Dementia's medical student lecture on Alzheimer's disease and other dementias. UCI Alzheimer's Disease Research Center. *http://uci.edu/differential.dx.html*; February 23.

# Not for the Elderly[2]

By Sanjay Gupta, M.D.
*Time*, December 24, 2001


A million American senior citizens each year take drugs they
should probably never be given. What to watch for

Something is wrong with the way drugs are prescribed to the elderly in this country. Every year, according to last week's *Journal of
the American Medical Association*, nearly 7 million older Americans—about one-fifth of the population age 65 or older—are given
medications that are rarely appropriate for people their age. Worse
still, the same article reports, nearly 1 million swallow pills that an
expert panel has determined senior citizens should probably never
take.

How does this happen? Mix-ups, pill sharing and people using
expired prescriptions contribute, but at least part of the problem is
the way doctors are trained. Pediatrics is mandatory in all U.S.
medical schools, but geriatric care tends to get glossed over. In pedi-
atric rotations, I was told over and over that kids are not little
adults. They are treated differently and get different drugs and dosages.

Not so the elderly. Seniors, despite appearances, are not just older
adults. The human body goes through changes as it ages, externally
and internally. The elderly often have less muscle mass, a slower
metabolism and greater sensitivity to certain drugs. Yet the recommended dosages for most medications are based on a 154-lb. man of
normal metabolism—with no allowance for age.

Case in point: propoxyphene (Darvon), which for the elderly offers
no better pain relief than aspirin or Tylenol and is known to be
addictive. Yet more than 6% of the seniors surveyed had been prescribed propoxyphene. Even more serious are a variety of modern
tranquilizers and hypnotics, such as flurazepam (Somnol) and chlor-
diazepoxide (Librium). These medicines can lead to falls and hip
fractures.

The most disturbing stories I've heard are from older patients who
complain to their doctors about the adverse effects of their medication and are told that they are "just getting old." The fault is not
always with the doctor, Dr. Arlene Bierman, one of the authors of
the study, is quick to add. "Physicians want to give good care, and
patients want to receive it," she says. But a situation that was
already bad is getting worse as the population ages and new medications proliferate.

There is also an underlying problem with our medical system that Dr. Jerry Avorn, writing in an accompanying editorial, describes as the "triumph of habit over evidence." Doctors tend to write the prescriptions they're used to writing, rather than boning up on the latest drugs.

There is talk of instituting technological fixes—pharmacy-based warning systems or handheld devices that give doctors up-to-date drug lists. An enhanced focus on geriatric care in medical school would also help, as would annual medication reviews. But for now, seniors may have to fend for themselves. They should never change prescriptions without consulting their physicians, but they should feel free to question their doctors if they find themselves taking medications from the list of drugs to avoid.

---

## Keep Away From . . .

**Flurazepam:**
Dalmane and Somnol, e.g.

**Meprobamate:**
Equanil, Meprospan, Miltown

**Chlorpropamide:**
Diabinese

**Meperidine:**
Demerol

**Pentazocine:**
Talwin

**Trimethobenzamide:**
Tigan, Benzacot, Stemetic

**Dicyclomine:**
Bentyl

**Hyoscyamine:**
Anaspaz, Cystospaz, Gastrosed

**Propantheline:**
Pro-Banthine

**Barbiturates:**
pentobarbital

**Belladonna Alkaloids:**
atropine

# The New "War against Aging"[3]

BY IRENE ALLEGER
*TOWNSEND LETTER FOR DOCTORS & PATIENTS*, JULY 1997

When I first read a few years ago of the formation of a new group of physicians and researchers to "combat aging," it made me uneasy. Now this concept is beginning to take on momentum, with all kinds of people getting on the bandwagon. In February the FDA announced that they want to "jumpstart" clinical research for a totally new category of pharmaceutical agents—"Anti-Aging Therapeutics." When you consider that the pharmaceutical conglomerates probably have whole departments that do nothing but watch trends and demographics, it becomes obvious that this may be the biggest "cash cow" they could ever hope for. We are rapidly becoming a population of "senior citizens"—a huge new market for a new class of drugs.

Our culture has never had much use for old age—a youthful appearance has been valued more than wisdom and experience. The hormonal steroids such as DHEA and melatonin are getting much of the attention so far as "youth extenders." But on the horizon are biotechnological interventions—genetic engineering, surgery, live cell therapy, more organ transplants, and of course, more drugs. However, the most questionable aspect of this new "war" is the subtle manipulation of turning degenerative diseases caused by faulty diet and environmental pollution, into "degenerative disorders of aging."

What is the difference between "the adverse effects of the aging process," and degenerative diseases caused by our modern diet and polluted environment? Doesn't everyone know by now that poor nutrition and pollution accelerate aging?

Nutritional science has proven conclusively that diet is crucial in preventing degenerative disease (and therefore extends life). Theoretically, if one could avoid all environmental pollutants and eat only wholesome, unprocessed food, one could not only live to a ripe old age, but enjoy a quality of life that cannot be obtained in any other way. Turning preventable, lifestyle-caused diseases into "aging," which can then be treated with new high-tech modalities and drugs, appears to be another end run by the drug companies. The focus on this new market will also slow progress on validating non-drug medicine, siphoning off funds for research on alternatives.

Our culture has so emphasized youth (because we're a relatively young country?) that we've developed a pathological denial of old age and death. Some of it may be caused by the misery of ill health and the specter of the nursing home that most Americans see in

---

their future today. But we know it doesn't have to be like that. Most of the centenarians I've read about have lived healthy lifestyles—they don't attribute their longevity to a new drug or medical intervention! In fact, most seem to have avoided drugs altogether.

The Anti-Aging group, in demanding "official recognition of aging as a treatable disorder," may have, in fact, opened the door to the pharmaceutical companies, and the FDA, to push more bad medicine onto the American public. The FDA: "Thousands of physicians practicing innovative medicine and their millions of patients suffering from the degenerative effects of aging, have been waiting for this news" (the patent holders for hormones certainly have been).

The idea of extending life is not new—hucksters have been selling immortality for centuries if not millennia. What is different now is that we have the technological ability to manipulate the human body in ways that were not imagined a few decades ago. We now start pumping drugs into 6-month old infants; manipulate conception and birth in a dozen different ways; transplant animal organs into humans; and have now let the genetic genie out of the bottle. From birth to death, we have become guinea pigs. Whether with pharmaceutical drugs, experimental surgery, or genetic engineering, we are in unknown territory, and I fear that our belief in technology is leading us into yet another dead end.

# Fountains of Youth[4]

BY SHARON BEGLEY
*NEWSWEEK*, FALL/WINTER 2001

Although researchers of earlier times never came close to cracking the secret of longevity, they were on the right track: to sustain the health and extend the lives of the old, you probably need to mine the essence of youth from the young. English scientists of the 13th century therefore believed that the breath of a virgin would rejuvenate old men, while a physiologist in 1920s Vienna theorized that elderly men would find renewed vigor and extra years by having the testicles of younger men grafted onto their original equipment. Neither approach, needless to say, worked. But today's researchers are thinking along the same lines. To replace and repair cells damaged by the diseases of aging, go to the youngest of the young: days-old human embryos.

A Four-Day Human embryo is a hollow ball of cells, no bigger than the dot over this i. Its inner layer contains the now famous embryonic stem cells—famous less for what they can do than for where they come from. Because stem cells come from "spare" embryos that fertility clinics intend to discard (because the would-be mother no longer needs them), the very idea of using them for medical research and treatment ignited a political firestorm pitting many right-to-life advocates against patients and their advocates. President George W. Bush's decision in August to prohibit federal funding for research using any but already existing cells (taken from embryos months or years ago and now growing in labs) pleased the right more than it did scientists and patients. He "may have compromised the science and delayed cures," warns Dr. Michael Soules, president of the American Society for Reproductive Medicine.

Stem cells offer the promise of cures because they have not yet decided what they will be when they grow up. They are "pluripotent," which means they have the potential to differentiate into any of the 200-plus cell types that make up a human body, from heart and liver cells to skin cells and neurons. What the cells actually become depends on which of their 30,000 or so genes (identical in every human cell) turn on. If genes characteristic of a cardiac-muscle cell turn on, while genes characteristic of all other cells remain turned off, then that stem grows up into a cell of the heart muscle. If genes characteristic of a dopamine-producing neuron turn on, then that stem cell is committed to becoming a dopamine-producing neuron.

---

4. From *Newsweek*, Fall/Winter 2001. © 2001 Newsweek, Inc. All rights reserved. Reprinted by permission.

In 1998, scientists discovered how to isolate and grow embryonic stem cells so that the cells maintain their pluripotency—that is, they remain a seemingly endless source of any kind of cell. The next step was to turn them into particular kinds of cells. And that has gone faster than anyone dreamed. By last December, scientists led by physiologist John D. Gearhart of Johns Hopkins University had figured out how to turn human embryonic stem

*The greatest hopes for stem cells center on their use in neurodegenerative diseases like Parkinson's and ALS.*

cells into 10 kinds of cells, including heart muscle, skin cells and T cells of the immune system. In June, they were up to 110. "We have the technology to make infinite quantities of all cellular tissue," says Dr. Thomas Okarma, CEO of Geron Corp.

And then what? Stem cells "may have the potential to generate replacement cells for a broad array of tissues and organs, such as the heart, the pancreas, and the nervous system," concluded a National Institutes of Health (NIH) report released in July. They thus hold the promise "of being able to repair or replace cells or tissues that are damaged or destroyed by . . . devastating diseases." It's called regenerative medicine. Stem cells might one day treat Parkinson's disease, chronic heart disease, rheumatoid arthritis and osteoarthritis, liver failure, diabetes, spinal-cord injury, multiple sclerosis. Okarma guesses that clinical trials are only three to five years away.

The greatest hopes for stem cells center on their use in neurodegenerative diseases like Parkinson's and ALS (amyotrophic lateral sclerosis, or Lou Gehrig's disease). Researchers hope to grow undifferentiated stem cells in a lab dish and nudge them into becoming the desired kind of neuron. Then, after drilling through the skull, a surgeon would implant the cells. This year Gearhart and colleagues showed, in rats, how it might work. They took human embryonic cells, induced them to start functioning like neurons and injected them into the fluid surrounding the injured spinal cords of rats. Three months later many of the once paralyzed rats could walk again. In rats paralyzed by a stroke in the motor cortex, stem cells also worked magic: transplanted into the brain, they seemed to mature into motor-cortex neurons. The rats could move again. Such new neurons might similarly help ALS patients.

In Parkinson's disease, dopamine-carrying neurons die. Fully developed dopamine neurons don't survive transplantation. An alternative, then, is to grow stem cells, coax them down the path toward becoming dopamine neurons, then implant them in the patient's brain, where they would (with any luck) grow, differentiate and link up to existing neurons. Ron McKay of NIH has now gotten mouse embryonic stem cells to start turning into dopamine neurons. When he implanted them in rats with the rodent version of Parkinson's, the characteristic tremor of the disease disappeared.

Stem cells might repair a broken heart, too. In August, researchers at the Technion-Israel Institute of Technology announced that they had induced human embryonic stem cells toward becoming heartmuscle cells, called cardiomyocytes. The next step is to grow the cells in huge quantities so that several million can be injected into a damaged heart. Since the shortage of donor hearts can otherwise be a death sentence, "this new research may lead to breakthrough tools" to treat cardiac disease, says Technion's Dr. Rafael Beyar.

In autoimmune diseases, the immune system mistakes the body's own cells for invaders and attacks them mercilessly. In rheumatoid arthritis, immune-system cells attack joints; in lupus, they attack skin, joints, the brain and kidneys; in multiple sclerosis, immune cells attack the myelin that coats neurons. Current treatments include anti-inflammatory drugs and immunosuppressants, but they are far from perfect. In stem-cell therapy, the patient's own immune-system cells would be destroyed, probably with radiation. They would be replaced, through a transfusion, with cells that had been produced by embryonic stem cells and that act as precursors of all immune-system cells. Presto: a new immune system that doesn't mistake self for invader. And to repair cartilage lost to rheumatoid arthritis, cartilage-building cells called chondrocytes, derived from stem cells, could then be transfused into the patient. Something comparable might be done to repair myelin lost to MS. Two years ago Harvard scientists used stem cells to repair the myelin in mice that had an MS-like disease.

The cause of Type I diabetes is well understood—the immune system destroys insulin-producing cells in the pancreas—but a cure has proved elusive. (A pancreas transplant helps some 80 percent of recipients, but there is a shortage of organs for transplant, and the lifetime of immunosuppressive drugs required makes patients vulnerable to infections and diseases, including cancer.) Last year researchers in Spain cultured stem cells in the lab and induced them to develop into the insulin-making islet cells. Implanted into the spleens of mice, the cells reversed the animals' symptoms of diabetes.

Bush is pushing for more studies of stem cells derived from adult tissue, since those pose no ethical dilemma. But adult stem cells do not proliferate as well as embryonic ones, which could be a problem when you need millions of cells for transplant. Because of the limits Bush placed on stem-cell research, regenerative medicine will likely arrive later than it otherwise might have. But if the paralyzed rats that walk again and the Parkinson's-beset rats that lose their tremors are harbingers, arrive it will.

# Long-Term Blues[5]

BY PAMELA SHERRID
*U.S. NEWS & WORLD REPORT*, MAY 27, 2002

In the insular world of nursing home executives, Terrance Kuzman has clout. He does a diligent job as administrator of the Parkway Pavilion, a 140-bed nursing home in Enfield, Conn. But Kuzman's special influence stems from a simple geographic fact: The facility he runs is located in the district of Rep. Nancy Johnson of Connecticut, who heads the House Ways and Means Committee's powerful subcommittee on health. Kuzman has kept Johnson abreast of his industry's problems for years and credits her for helping to soften the various blows imposed by federal budget cutters on the $96 billion nursing home industry.

It will be a busy summer for Kuzman and other members of his industry's grass-roots lobbying army. The current wrangling over the federal budget carries high stakes for the nation's 17,000 nursing homes, about two thirds of which are for-profit. The industry is just emerging from a period of intense woe in which three of the five major for-profit nursing home chains filed for bankruptcy, even as they were under pressure to improve the quality of care. A significant factor in the industry's downfall was severe cuts in Medicare spending that began taking their toll in 1998. Thanks in part to Congress's rolling back some of those cuts, most of the chains have recently emerged from bankruptcy. But that $1.8 billion giveback is due to expire in September, giving tremendous urgency to this year's budget battle.

There's a sad irony in the nursing-home industry's focus on Medicare, the nation's health insurance program for seniors. While only 10 percent to 15 percent of nursing home residents are Medicare patients, Medicare provides 25 percent of nursing home revenue. (Medicare typically pays only if a patient's stay follows a three-day hospitalization and then only for 100 days of care.) The bulk of nursing home patients are on Medicaid, the state-federal program for the poor.

This is a case of the few paying for the many. According to a recent industry study, Medicare payments earn homes a rich margin of more than 20 percent. But that profit is many nursing homes' lifeblood because Medicaid in most states doesn't pay enough to cover the costs of caring for the old, sick, and frail. "We lose money on 75 percent of our patients," says Kuzman.

---

While Medicare pays Parkway Pavilion $300 a day for each Medicare patient, Medicaid pays $128 a day, $9 below its cost. The nursing home industry says a $9-a-day deficit is typical, amounting to a $3.7 billion shortfall for the industry annually. In Wisconsin, an $11-a-day-per-patient shortfall recently prompted nonprofit Lincoln Lutheran Care Center to announce the closure of one of its three facilities in the Racine area. Like some other nonprofits, Lincoln Lutheran has an endowment, but it's "just not big enough to cover our losses," says its CEO, the Rev. Daniel Risch.

The situation is exacerbated by the fact that many middle-class people who could pay for their own nursing home care believe they shouldn't have to. Guided by aggressive estate-planning lawyers, aging parents shift assets to their heirs so the parents can go on Medicaid if long-term care proves necessary later on. "We see families do that all the time," says Risch.

**Empty Wallets**

The patients who do foot their own bills typically pay more than the Medicaid rate. (At Parkway Pavilion, private patients pay $200 a day.) Many become impoverished and eventually go on Medicaid. So far, few people have bought long-term-care insurance, so the roster of private payers hasn't increased much as a result. And nursing homes have seen private-pay revenue dry up because of another trend: the boom in assisted-living facilities that lure seniors who might otherwise have opted for a nursing home.

| Coming Back from the Brink | |
| --- | --- |
| **Score Card:** The United States has 1.8 million nursing home beds. The top five providers are all for-profit chains. After a few disastrous years, the industry is trying to regain its footing. | |
| **Nursing Home** | **Beds** |
| **Beverly Enterprises:** New management is improving profits and looking for growth. | 51,000 |
| **Manor Care:** Most profitable chain; large proportion of private payers. | 41,200 |
| **Kindred Healthcare (formerly Vencor):** Emerged from bankruptcy in 2001, entered in 1999. | 38,000 |
| **Mariner Post-Acute Network:** Emerged from bankruptcy this month, entered in 2000. | 37,400 |
| **Genesis Health Ventures:** Emerged from bankruptcy in 2001, entered in 2000. | 33,000 |

Source: The American Health Care Association

There are undeniable political risks for nursing homes in trumpeting the fact that Medicare is subsidizing Medicaid. "Until recently, nursing homes never wanted to come out and say that Medicare was overpaying them," says Thomas Scully, administrator of the federal Centers for Medicare & Medicaid Services. The independent federal agency that advises Congress on Medicare, known as MedPAC, made it clear in January that it feels Congress should allow the givebacks to expire. "Our commissioners don't believe Medicare should be the tail wagging the [Medicaid] dog," says Sally Kaplan, MedPAC's research director for post-acute care. In the aftermath, nursing home stocks fell 17 percent, though most have since recovered on hopes that Congress will answer the industry's pleas.

Nursing home lobbyists would, of course, like to see Medicaid payments raised. But to them, maintaining Medicare rates seems a more practical short-term goal. State governments are under

---

*"Until recently, nursing homes never wanted to come out and say that Medicare was overpaying them."*—Thomas Scully, **Centers for Medicare & Medicaid Services**

---

intense budget pressure because of the recent recession, and fast-growing Medicaid costs are often their second-largest expense after education. Indiana actually cut its Medicaid rates to nursing homes recently, and many other states are considering cuts or freezes. "Right now, Medicare is the only game in town," says John Schaeffler, chief lobbyist for the American Health Care Association, a nursing home trade group.

As they make their calls on Capitol Hill in the coming months, nursing home advocates will be rubbing elbows with lobbyists from other medical providers, such as doctors and hospitals, all looking for a fatter piece of the Medicare pie. Changes in payments to one group of providers reverberates on other groups. For instance, hospitals' tendency to discharge patients "quicker and sicker" because of flat fees from Medicare means that nursing homes have higher costs caring for those patients.

Now the Bush administration has intensified the competition by suggesting that any Medicare increases for one provider group be balanced by reductions for another. The early bets are that doctors, howling from a recent Medicare rate cut, will get their wish—at the expense of hospitals. But the 900-pound gorilla dominating Medicare talks this year is the desire of politicians to give seniors an expensive new benefit—prescription drug coverage.

The nursing home bargaining position is also weakened by the industry's own flaws. The companies that succumbed to bankruptcy in 1999 and 2000 made their own mistakes and can't blame government spending cuts for all their troubles. Though it seems unlikely now, in the early and mid-'90s nursing home chains were Wall Street darlings. They spent vast sums acquiring more facilities and other service providers to bump up lucrative Medicare revenues that were later cut back. "In retrospect, we paid too much for acquisitions," says Michael Walker, CEO of Genesis Health Ventures.

## Quality Control

Of course, poor patient care, from bedsores to sexual abuse, has long harmed the industry's reputation. Last month the federal government unveiled quality report cards on individual nursing homes that measure, among other things, the percentage of patients with weight loss, pain, and bedsores. "Some nursing homes are a little flipped out" by the initiative, says CMS's Scully. "But many in the industry are convinced they need quality improvement to get sympathy from Washington and state capitals."

Meanwhile, there is new management at several of the big chains. Beverly Enterprises, the largest for-profit nursing home operator with 466 homes in 28 states, escaped bankruptcy, but its new CEO, William Floyd, is a rookie in the industry, having served in top roles at Choice Hotels and Taco Bell. "Those businesses have more in common with nursing homes than you'd imagine," says Floyd. "They all involve managing many locations with thin margins." What's more, Taco Bell and nursing homes compete for the same low-wage workers.

Floyd has jettisoned Beverly's homes in Florida, where lawyers have found that suing the industry makes them rich. He's also closing laggard homes, shuttering wings in low-occupancy homes, and strengthening management. And Beverly is converting facilities specifically for Alzheimer's patients as the demand for such care mounts.

Still, there's no denying the industry's dependence on government coffers. And while adequate funding does not guarantee quality of care, it certainly plays a role. If Congress chooses to reduce funding, the impact will not be as bad as it was in the past decade because the nursing home companies are not as heavily burdened with debt. But Merrill Lynch predicts Beverly's earnings will fall by 16 percent, and Moody's recently sounded an alert about the bonds of Good Samaritan, the largest nonprofit chain.

No matter the outcome of the current Medicare debate, the financial health of the industry remains precarious. "Long-term care needs a long-term solution," says Robert Kane, a gerontologist at the Minnesota School of Public Health. "Right now we are keeping the bus rolling with spit and bailing wire."

# Dying in Peace[6]

By Wendy Murray Zoba
*Christianity Today*, October 22, 2001

As I arrived at the Balm of Gilead, a palliative-care unit on the fourth floor of Cooper Green Hospital in Birmingham [AL], one of the nurses was blowing her nose. Arnold Smith (not his real name) died that morning. Three nurses had gathered behind the nurse's station. "When people die, it is not unusual to find the leadership team in the nurse's station in a huddle, crying and praying," says Edwina Taylor, R.N., nurse practitioner and go-to person at Balm of Gilead. "Our faith holds us up."

Palliative care is not hospice care, though the two can easily be confused. Hospice care typically takes place in the dying person's home, or in a home-like setting. According to the National Hospice Foundation (NHF), it is a team-oriented approach of medical care, pain management, and spiritual support that is tailored to the patient's needs and wishes. Hospice care, the NHF says, upholds "the belief that each of us has the right to die pain-free and with dignity."

The same can be said of palliative care, with a notable difference: through pain and symptom control, palliative care readies dying patients to move from impersonal institutional settings into the gentler environment of hospice care whether at their home, in a nursing facility, or, if necessary, in the palliative-care unit itself. Dr. Amos Bailey, Balm of Gilead's former medical director, highlights the point that "75 percent of the people who die in the United States die in medical institutions." Fifty percent die in hospitals, another 25 percent in nursing homes. These "institutional" deaths are often painful, lonely, and isolated.

Palliative care is trying to change that picture. One might think of it as the meeting ground between hospice and institutional medical care. Situated on-site in a hospital, a palliative-care unit is a clearinghouse of sorts through which dying patients in the hospital, who have not received hospice care, get their symptoms stabilized and are then released from the hospital to die—not lonely, isolated deaths, but in a more personal, compassionate setting. Once patients have been through a palliative-care unit like Balm of Gilead, they are channeled seamlessly into the care of a local hospice.

---

6. Article by Wendy Murray Zoba from *Christianity Today* October 22, 2001. Copyright © Wendy Murray Zoba. Reprinted with permission.

Balm of Gilead refers terminally ill patients from all parts of Cooper Green Hospital—patients with AIDS, cancer, cirrhosis of the liver, heart and lung failure—to one of the 15 area hospices in Birmingham. Palliative care is still up-and-coming, but more medical institutions are recognizing its merit. Like hospice, it "addresses physical, spiritual, social, and emotional suffering through symptom control in those four areas for people who have a disease that man cannot cure," says Edwina Taylor, and it makes hospice care an option for more and more patients who might otherwise die alone in a sterile hospital bed."

## Communication Breakdown

Despite the soon-to-double number of aging Americans, most don't want to think or talk about how to die. There are now 40 million elderly people in the United States. In the next 30 years, with the aging of the baby boomers, that number will double. One third of those 80 million deaths will involve a chronic illness of some sort. Every chronic illness will require decisions, either on the part of the patient or the family. If present trends persist, most of these people will not have thought through end-of-life questions.

According to a national survey taken by the National Hospice Federation in April 1999, Americans are more likely to talk to their children about drugs and sex than about how they want to die.

- One in four people are not likely to discuss death-related issues with their aging parents, even if a parent is terminally ill and has less than six months to live.

- Fewer than 25 percent of Americans have thought about how they would like to be cared for at the end of life and have put it in writing.

- 36 percent say they have told someone about how they want to receive treatment at the end of life, but people include "passing comments" in this category. Even so, 50 percent of Americans overwhelmingly say they will rely on family and friends to make end-of-life decisions.

- Nearly 80 percent of Americans do not think of hospice as a choice for end-of-life care; 75 percent do not know that hospice care can be provided at home; fewer than 10 percent know that hospice provides pain relief for the terminally ill; more than 90 percent of Americans do not know that hospice care is a fully covered Medicare benefit.

The NHF calls it a national "communications challenge."

Hospice care has come a long way since its inauspicious beginnings in the late 1950s in Britain. More than 40 years later, 3,000 programs have been launched in the United States and more than 450,000 patients have sought hospice rare in their last stages of life.

Making more people aware of the benefits of hospice care has been a challenge. The medical establishment excels at curing people and is hard-pressed to surrender to death, which smacks of failure. This reticence also sometimes leaves patients ill-equipped to face their final days. A recent study conducted by the University of Chicago found that nearly 40 percent of the 258 doctors surveyed said they "would knowingly give inaccurate estimate of survival time, even if the patient had specifically asked for a frank prediction. Most doctors erred on the side of optimism" (*Chicago Tribune*, June 19). But beyond institutional resistance, the pragmatic youth-oriented culture we live in also works against having this conversation.

Balm of Gilead is among the first palliative-care units in the nation trying to change the tide. And only Balm of Gilead has worked with local Christian churches and other religious groups to help make it work. The small cadre of pioneers on Cooper Green's fourth floor are linking the medical establishment with the hospice movement and inviting religious believers to join in. More and more, Balm of Gilead and other palliative-care units are getting those 75 percent of patients destined to die in impersonal institutions into the hands of someone who cares about their pain, their families, and their spiritual life. Like the words of the black spiritual for which it is named, Balm of Gilead stands behind this truth: "There is a balm in Gilead that makes the wounded whole."

*The medical establishment excels at curing people and is hard-pressed to surrender to death, which smacks of failure.*

## A Rebel Movement

Amos Bailey notes that hospice care was "an antiphysician movement" in its beginnings. In the 1940s a British "almoner," or patient's advocate, named Cicily Saunders (now Dame Cicily) had witnessed the difficult isolated deaths of terminally ill patients, and her heart was moved. She felt a calling to serve and help them. She spoke to a trusted friend, a physician, who told her, "Go study medicine. It is the doctors who desert the dying." She completed her medical degree in 1957 at the age of 39, and after much prayer and meditation came up with a plan. St. Christopher's Hospice was born in 1967 in a London suburb, and with it the hospice movement.

Those renegade beginnings account for some of the languid response to hospice by the medical establishment. "Physicians and traditional [medical personnel] weren't paying attention to those who were dying," says Bailey. "They weren't very involved and were happy not to be involved, at least initially. It was primarily nurses and other support people who were dissatisfied with the kind of care that dying people were receiving. In reaction to that, they decided they didn't want to be in hospitals. Cicily Saunders

## Hospice Care Underused

PEOPLE'S MEDICAL SOCIETY NEWSLETTER, APRIL 2002

When should you consider hospice care? That's one of the many decisions and concerns that must be addressed when someone is dealing with advanced illness. A hospice, as you may already know, is a special facility designed solely to assist dying patients and their families.

Hospice care places emphasis on providing comfort and relief from symptoms, preparation for death and support for survivors. Care can be provided in the home or in professional, facilities with a home-like setting, but tile idea is to allow death with dignity and keep the family close to the patient, away from the high-tech surroundings of a hospital. In fact, the active contributions and support of family members are welcomed.

According to various studies and surveys, use of hospice services is on the increase. No surprise there, given the aging population and the fact that Medicare now provides for hospice coverage both in arid out of the home, but it's also true that more people with terminal conditions could be helped by the comprehensive set of services provided in hospice care. Joanne Lynn, M.D., director of the RAND Center to Improve Care of the Dying, says that too often doctors think only to recommend hospice care to people with cancer (January 2002 *Consumer Reports on Health*). Fact is, people with other advanced diseases, such as Alzheimer's or heart disease, should consider hospice.

Back to our original question of when, in the course of terminal illness: Most experts agree that if a persons life expectancy is six months or less, hospice care might be of value.

For help in dealing with advanced illness and its attendant issues—such as spiritual and emotional concerns, hospice, funeral planning and advanced medical planning—take a look at a Web site created at Michigan State University: *www.completingalife.msu.edu*.

What about other sources, such as hospice organizations? There are several throughout the country, some with, their own specialties, such as terminally ill children. These groups can provide you with a wealth of information on care for the terminally ill, as well as put you in touch with support groups. help you with Medicare reimbursement issues, and refer you to homemaker-health aides.

The following is a partial list of resources on this issue:

• Children's Hospice International, 703-684-0330

• Hospice Foundation of America, 800-854-3402

• National Association for Homecare, 202-546-4759

• National Hospice and Palliative Care Organization, 703-243-5900 or 800-658-8898

opened a residential unit [in a hospital]. But we don't have very many of those in the United States. We have primarily home hospice programs."

But the hospice movement's "antiphysician" roots explain only part of the medical profession's sluggishness. The starting point for hospice care is the abandonment of hope for recovery. This starkly contradicts a medical institution's curative approach. "Physicians see a dying patient as a defeat, like they didn't do their job," says Edwina Taylor. "They emotionally withdraw from them."

Adds Bailey, "People [in the medical community] feel powerless and don't know what to do. Studies have been done where they put cameras in front of the doors of rooms of patients who were dying. As the person got sicker, fewer people went in. And when they went in, they stayed for shorter periods of time. It's very uncomfortable. If they can't help this person, then being in the room with them and spending time with them is unpleasant. They don't want to be in that situation."

Hospice and palliative care—in addition to managing physical symptoms—also rally around the emotional, social, and spiritual aspects of dying, areas for which the medical community has not presumed expertise. Bailey, Taylor, the small Balm of Gilead staff, and their army of volunteers are making the case to the medical establishment that all of these aspects are essential to the human condition and need to be integrated into the dying process.

## Lessons from "the Last Hours"

Birmingham has been called "the Pittsburgh of the South," an old rust-bowl steel town with a high unemployment rate and lots of people on welfare who can't afford medical coverage. Early in my visit, I chatted with Miss Sunday, an African-American nurse sitting behind the glass encircling the nurse's station. Behind her on the window are sunny images of flowers, bumblebees, and trees. A sign reads: IT'S SPRINGTIME AT THE BALM OF GILEAD. She is a jolly dumpling of a woman who tells me, "We don't hear about many [dying] people who have loved ones at home. They really need help and don't have a clue where to get it from." The majority of terminal patients who come to Balm of Gilead, 70 percent, are minorities and poor. Many don't have health insurance.

Miss Sunday hands me a chart. It lists the churches that sponsor rooms at Balm of Gilead. Her church, Faith Apostolic, sponsors Room 417. That means church members set up the room with cozy furniture, including a comfortable sleeping chair for family, and a TV/VCR (about $5,000). They also oversee the steady flow of volunteers who water the flowers, put together care packages for the patients, play the guitar and sing, or sit and hold the hands of the dying in Room 417. The sponsoring church or community group "owns" a room. There are ten such rooms at Balm of Gilead that serve approximately 200 patients a year.

Miss Sunday is one of a paid team of five at Balm of Gilead, which has no secretary or copy machine. She is a busy person. They all are busy in that hallway. I thank her for her time. "We're happy to entertain, mmm hmm," she says.

About an hour later, I am sitting off to the side in a meeting room on Cooper Green's eighth floor. Medical students, interns, and residents have gathered around the meeting table for the "Morning

Report." Their shirts and ties are hidden under white coats and green surgical outfits. They have stethoscopes around their necks. Some are sipping Pepsi or coffee from mugs.

These doctors and doctors-in-training receive four 15-minute sessions daily from various specialists who work at the hospital. I am sitting in on Bailey's session. It is up to him to help these students get their heads around this notion of holistic end-of-life care. Most will not know what palliative care is. Medical schools do not teach it. Today's discussion is called "The Last Hours of Life."

"Mr. Smith has small-cell lung cancer. He is in the active dying process," Bailey begins. "What are the symptoms of someone who is actively dying?"

There is a flurry of response:

"Pain."

"Secretion."

"Dyspnea."

"Drying of the membranes, eye and mouth."

"Depression."

Bailey is discussing what a doctor can do for a patient who has entered the active dying process. He is trying to help these students understand that doctors do not have to throw up their arms, shut the door, and walk away from a dying patient. "Doctors write orders," he tells them. "I want you to be able to write orders better."

Bailey is an Episcopalian who wears a bow tie with earthy cottons, reads *Sojourners*, and speaks in soft, measured intonations. He is a kind man, unharried by the unrelenting demands foisted upon him from students, interns, and residents, as well as the dying. He is strongly fixed on his sense of calling. He lives to relieve the suffering of dying people.

He was born and raised in rural Florida, the first of his family to graduate from high school. He put himself through college on an accelerated schedule and knew he wanted to go to medical school, though he couldn't decide between psychiatry and internal medicine. He chose the latter, with a specialty in hematology and subspecialty in oncology. He completed a fellowship at the University of Alabama at Birmingham (UAB), where he caught his first glimpse of the serious gap that existed between medical care and the treatment of the dying. "I saw lots of unrelieved suffering and didn't have a clue about what to do about it," he says.

Upon completing his training, he moved to Appalachia, in West Virginia, where he practiced internal medicine and oncology among the rural poor. "Everything I learned about palliative care, I learned from those experiences," he says. Self-taught, he gained firsthand training in end-of-life care and became the medical director of a hospice that served low-income mountain people, bringing to bear all aspects of well-being (emotional, social, and spiritual with the physical) to his medical care. Many of his patients were homebound, so he began making house calls, a practice that he continues today. He also stepped into the void among physicians willing to treat patients with HIV.

Bailey returned in 1994 to the UAB'S Cooper Green Hospital, where he now practices as a medical oncologist and supervises medical students and residents. He is Alabama's first board-certified physician for hospice and palliative care, and he was recently elected to the Fellowship of the American College of Physicians. Married and the father of three, he builds birdhouses his daughter designs when he is not training the residents or adjusting the MSConcentrate levels of the dying.

Morning Report participants had no difficulty rattling off the symptoms that attend active dying. Knowing how to best serve the patient was more of a challenge. Bailey drew a road map. Doctors can actively treat and participate in the dying process of a patient,

---

*Doctors can actively treat and participate in the dying process of a patient, . . . and there is a way of doing it that hands patients the controls and helps and comforts them.*

---

he wants them to understand, and there is a way of doing it that hands patients the controls and helps and comforts them. "We want to get away from IVs, NG tubes, restraints, oxygen masks, and isolation from family," he says. "There is a way of treating Mr. Smith that doesn't use these things. These really don't help people."

He goes back over the list of symptoms. For Mr. Smith's pain, "we decided not to use MSContin and use MSConcentrate instead. It goes under the tongue, so he doesn't have to swallow." It helps Mr. Smith to take medication that dissolves under the tongue.

"For the secretions, we put a Scopolamine patch behind his ear. That gets rid of the death rattle [a gurgling sound produced by mucus in the lungs of a dying person]. The death rattle, actually, is more of a concern for the family than the patient. It is very uncomfortable to listen to. It drives families away." Scopolamine helps Mr. Smith not to drive his family away.

"For the Dyspnea [labored breathing], an $O^2$ nasal prong, as tolerated, as he wants it." Mr. Smith determines how much he can tolerate.

"For the drying of the membranes of the eyes, we can give him saline eye drops. You can assign this to the families. They want to do things." It helps Mr. Smith and his family to participate in his care.

"Depression is often associated with the family. Yesterday, in the throes of death, Mr. Smith was holding on to see his daughter one last time. But she refused to come. She didn't want to see him dying. We had a chaplain come." Mr. Smith's pain was eased by caregivers who recognized his need for spiritual, as well as physical, care.

> *Controlling physical symptoms is only the beginning of palliative care.*

Bailey concludes his 15-minute presentation with an appeal for the students to read "Gone from My Sight," a booklet that outlines for patients and family what to expect in the last stages of death. "It only takes a few minutes to read. Families will read it over and over again. Hospice workers have put this together over many years. It is very reassuring to the patients and families if you know what they're concerned about and bring it up. It shows expertise on your part. It shows concern."

He lingers after the session to chat with students. "It was an incredible flail, trying to get his feeding tube down," one student says of a patient. "He goes in and out a lot." Bailey tells that student, "If he's delirious, just give him at least one scheduled dose."

We are walking down the hall on our way back to the fourth floor and Barley is stopped constantly in the hallway. I feel like I'm in the presence of a rock star. Students are lined up to speak with him. He looks at the chart one student presents to him. "You've got this right, but that wrong," he says.

(Since my visit to Balm of Gilead last spring, Bailey's role has changed. Though he still instructs students at the center, the program's success has given him the chance to develop a new palliative care unit at the nearby VA hospital. The program launches in January.)

**A Heart's Cry**

Controlling physical symptoms is only the beginning of palliative care. "We actually think that one of the worst deaths people can have is spiritual, when people are in spiritual anguish," Bailey says to me as we sit in his office. "We had a guy who was having nightmares about the fact that his family was religious and he wasn't. He had had a problem in his marriage and felt unforgiven. He said he wanted to be baptized. We arranged for a minister to come up who told him he could be sprinkled. But he wanted to be completely immersed. They were a Baptist family. So we filled a bathtub and let the minister baptize him.

"We had somebody who died this last week who was afraid of dying. I asked her what she thought happened to people when they die and she said, 'I think you just stop being.' She had lived a wild life. Then she became ill and started going to church. She tried to believe. But it was impossible for her to feel reassured by that. It caused tremendous struggle, hollering, and twitching."

"It was awful," adds Taylor. "It went on for days. We gave her very potent medicine to try and calm her down. She felt a little calmer but never got peaceful. Her life was just horrible, apparently. She had so much that was unresolved, it all came back to haunt her on her deathbed."

Taylor's defining color is red: her short, smartly clipped hair is red; so are her flowing knit dress, apple-shaped earrings, and lipstick. The color sets off her brilliant eyes, which shine when she smiles and when she cries. If Bailey embodies the gentle calm of symptom management and compassionate care, Taylor is the fire that bums in the heart of Balm of Gilead. Her "heart cry" is that no person dies alone and unresolved.

Later in my visit, we are sitting in her small, cramped office. Her desk is covered with papers and books and family photos of her two grown children. "When a person dies, it takes a whole lot of pulling together," she says. She outlines for me, in four aspects, how this heart cry plays out in that hallway.

The first is what she calls the power of presence. "Write that in Second Coming headlines," she says to me. "You don't abandon people. Nobody wants to die alone. Jesus said, 'Lo, I am with you always.' There is nothing greater than that. You don't have to say anything profound. There aren't enough profound things to say. But if you don't have to suffer alone, you can kind of do it."

Second, *affirmation of family*. Integrating family members into the dying process is critical. It allows the dying person to find resolution and release, in order to leave this world in peace. But bringing family into it can be "very messy," she says. "When a terminal illness occurs, all the problems in the family are magnified a thousand times. It is very difficult. We have families who haven't spoken for years. So we're treating the patient's symptoms, while working with the families all at the same time. It's like the Nike thing: You just do it. You don't do it right all the time. But you have to do it."

Third, *explain, explain, explain*. "We had a difficult death last week. I told the same story 16 times." The pain and shock of watching a loved one die leaves a family disoriented. Being willing to explain what's going on over and over again, she says, "enables people to move through the grieving."

Bailey told me about a patient who, in the months preceding death, was in and out of Balm of Gilead for an array of symptom-control problems. One of the complicating factors was the family, which for a long time refused to accept the gravity of her condition. It took repeated, often painful, conversations with Bailey before family members could come to terms with how to help their loved one.

At one point the patient was having trouble swallowing because of multiple strokes: "She couldn't swallow and had a feeding tube and kept getting congestive heart failure," Bailey says. "They would try to get rid of too much fluid, and then she'd have renal failure. Then they'd give her more fluid. It was flail back and forth, back and forth. Every time she'd come in, the house staff would say, 'Dr. Bailey, you have to talk to this family.' I'd go talk to them and they would be angry and yell at me and say, 'She's not really dying. She'll live.' They wouldn't accept it. I would go back a couple of months later and we would start the conversation again. Eventually they took her home and, eventually, she died peacefully. We just have to be sticking with her."

Being vigilant in explaining, Taylor says, "signals the family that you know what you are doing and that you are doing everything you can to relieve the suffering of their loved one." Often in the "explaining" stage she finds the opportunity to introduce a spiritual witness. She said to a mother whose son died of AIDS, "God knows how you feel. He watched his Son suffer and die, too."

*Nationally, only 15 percent of Americans take advantage of palliative care or hospice services.*

Fourth, *physical and emotional touch*. "We can touch people at some point in the human experience that we hold in common," she says. "I don't do boundaries." She told me about a crack addict they had in the hallway who was unruly and difficult, someone they all had to buck up to care for. As she drew near to death, they heard her say, "I think I'm going to die. I need to go to the bank to get money to buy shoes for my baby." This window into her soul opened up for the beleaguered staff a new compassion for this woman. "God is here," Taylor says. "He gives us his mercies and grace every day."

The phone rings. It is a worker from a local hospice calling to check on a breast-cancer patient at Balm of Gilead. Edwina tells the caller, "Well, she's not out dancin' in the halls, but she's not screamin' either." She put the receiver on the desk and went to check on the patient while the caller waited. After she hung up, Taylor told me the breast-cancer patient "will have to go into a nursing home, but hospice will follow her there."

### Going Home

Some have wondered if hospice, being a Medicare benefit, might open up greater possibilities to legalize physician-assisted suicide (PAS) to keep costs down. Bailey demurs. "People who have primarily availed themselves of this are white, middle-to-upper-class educated men, who have the illusion that they are in control—women and minorities and poorer people learned the lesson long ago that they're not in control. It is almost never because of poorly controlled symptoms. If anything, [PAS] has spurred the improvement in symptom management and pain control and the attention given to the dying.

"This is not rocket science," he says. "But people don't know about it." Several institutions have shown an interest in developing palliative-care programs and representatives from a number of Alabama hospitals have visited Balm of Gilead. It was also featured in a four-part Bill Moyers PBS special called *On Their Own Terms*, and there is an increasing literature available about how hospitals can introduce it into their programs.

Balm of Gilead is supported by a number of organizations, including the Robert Wood Johnson Foundation's Initiative for Excellence in End-of-Life Care, Cooper Green Hospital, and the Jefferson County Department of Health. It also has partnerships with local foundations, colleges and universities, faith communities, and civic and professional groups. Between November 1998, when Balm of Gilead opened, and July 2000, 347 patients died at Cooper Green Hospital. Of those, 180 (nearly 52 percent) had been moved to the palliative-care unit. Nationally, only 15 percent of Americans take advantage of palliative care or hospice services.

"People don't have to have crummy end-of-life care," says Bailey. "It's like the physician that doesn't know what to do. Well, patients and families don't know what to do either. And no one is there to help them, so they just muddle along. That's why people end up in ICU, when what they really need is to spend time in a room where their family can be with them.

"People think that to die you need a good doctor, a good nurse, a good social worker, a good chaplain, and maybe a good mental-health worker," he says. "I don't want to downplay that, but quite frankly, what people need is to stay connected with their community and their families. Instead, we take somebody who gets too sick to stay home and pluck them out of bed and put them someplace where you can only visit them a couple hours a day. And even that is not convenient, because it is during working hours when nobody can get there." (Balm of Gilead has no limits, for persons or hours, on visitation.)

"You've taken them out of their community and want 'professionals' to care for them when what people really want is to be with their family. The medical system does a terrible job. It doesn't know what to do.

"Professional caregivers can help, but this is something bigger. What people really need when they are facing death are five things: To say, 'I forgive you. Please forgive me. I love you. Thank you. Goodbye.'"

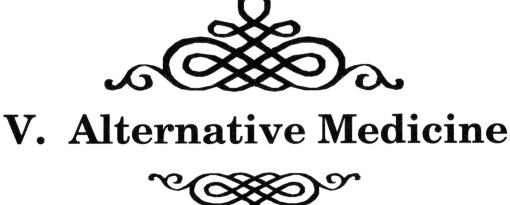

# V. Alternative Medicine

# Editor's Introduction

A growing mistrust of Western medicine and conventional practices has prompted many people to turn to alternative treatments and therapies, several of which are featured in chapter 5. From acupuncture to chiropractic to homeopathic remedies, these alternative treatments once considered fads are now becoming mainstream. Despite the growing popularity and respectability of alternative medicine, many traditional doctors still view it as a joke; they consider the so-called "specialists" in the field "quacks" and do not give their findings much credit. Meanwhile, a number of those in the alternative medical field think Western doctors are poisoning their patients by treating every ailment with some form of drug. Nevertheless, some practitioners on both sides are beginning to consider that traditional Western medicine and the new alternative techniques could be used in conjunction to treat their patients.

There are seven different classifications under the heading of alternative medicine. The first article in this section from the *World Almanac and Book of Facts* briefly explains these classifications and provides an overview of what each one entails. The remaining articles examine a few types of alternative therapies in greater detail by explaining how each treatment works, where it originated, and what it costs.

One form of alternative medicine which is meant to relieve pain is chiropractic. Between 15 and 20 million Americans visit chiropractors every year to treat back and neck pain. Once seen as a highly questionable practice, chiropractic is now widely accepted within the medical community and is even prescribed by some medical doctors. "Fact and Fiction About Chiropractic" describes the origins of this treatment, its growing support and acceptance over the years, its benefits and potential dangers, and how to choose a chiropractor.

Though not as accepted among the medical community as chiropractic, acupuncture has gained support among many Americans. Acupuncture involves reducing pain and treating ailments in certain parts of the body by inserting needles into specific areas, usually a quarter of an inch to one inch beneath the skin. Originating in China, acupuncture is believed to restore the body's Qi (or flow of energy) while relieving pain and discomfort. According to an article from *Monkeyshines on Health & Science*, this type of treatment is believed to be most beneficial to those with nervous and muscular system problems.

An altogether different treatment from chiropractic or acupuncture, homeopathy does not just focus on the physical aspects of healing; it diagnoses illness through observing mental and emotional symptoms as well. In "A Healthy Balance," Maria Rabat explains that, after an initial visit to a homeopathic practitioner (which usually runs two hours), a single-ingredient remedy is prescribed to treat the individual's ailment. The kinds of remedies prescribed are diluted plant, mineral, chemical, or animal-based substances. The more diluted the remedy, the more potent it is believed to be. This type of treatment is inexpensive and easy to administer, and there is little risk to the patient. This is perhaps why it is becoming so popular.

Herbal medicine, a treatment used since ancient times, resembles homeopathy in that it employs natural and organic substances to treat different ailments. In his article "Herbal Medicine: Use with Caution and Respect," Brian T. Sanderoff warns, "The notion that because a substance is 'natural' or 'comes from nature,' it cannot cause harm is false." He acknowledges the benefits of several herbal treatments but notes that different compounds affect the body in different ways. Since each of these remedies is composed of a different compound, Sanderoff asserts that people must consider how their bodies might react to an herbal remedy, which can cause anything from sickness to death if administered to someone with the wrong body type or in the wrong dosage.

Each of these articles emphasizes that alternative treatments are not the be-all and end-all of medical treatment. They stress that a medical doctor should be consulted in cases of severe or recurring symptoms.

# Alternative Medicine[1]

*WORLD ALMANAC & BOOK OF FACTS*, 2002

Alternative medicine comprises a wide variety of healing philosophies, approaches, and therapies. It includes treatments and health care practices not widely taught in medical schools, not generally used in hospitals, and not usually reimbursed by health insurance companies. The NIH cautions people not to seek alternative therapies without the consultation of a licensed health care provider.

Some alternative therapies are described as holistic—meaning that the practitioner considers the whole person, including physical, mental, emotional, and spiritual aspects. Some therapies are known as preventive, meaning that the practitioner stresses preventing health problems before they arise.

People may use an alternative therapy alone, along with other alternative therapies, or in combination with more standard therapies. Worldwide, only about 10–30% of health care is provided by conventional practitioners; the remaining 70–90% involves alternative practices. An estimated 1 in 3 Americans uses some form of alternative medicine.

An advisory panel to the National Center for Complementary and Alternative Medicine (formerly called the Office of Alternative Medicine) at the National Institutes of Health classified 7 general fields of practice:

Alternative systems of medical practice range from self-care based on folk traditions to care given by practitioners according to established procedures. Included are such therapies as acupuncture, Ayurveda (India's traditional system of natural medicine), environmental medicine (treatment of certain illnesses believed to be caused by exposure to particular foods or chemicals), homeopathic medicine (use of remedies made from naturally occurring plant, animal, or mineral substances), Native American practices, naturopathic medicine (integration of traditional, natural therapeutics with modern scientific medicine), and traditional Oriental medicine.

Bioelectromagnetic applications explore how living things interact with electromagnetic fields. Such therapies include blue light treatment and artificial lighting, electroacupuncture, and electrostimulation.

---

1. Article from *World Almanac & Book of Facts 2002*. Copyright © 2002 World Almanac Education Group, Inc. Reprinted with permission.

Diet, nutrition, and lifestyle changes are intended to prevent illness, maintain good health, and reverse the effects of chronic disease. Examples include use of macrobiotics, nutritional supplements, and megavitamins.

Herbal medicine employs plants and plant products for pharmacological use. Some common plants used are echinacea, garlic, ginkgo biloba, ginseng, St. John's wort, and saw palmetto.

Manual healing uses touch and manipulation with the hands therapeutically. Some types are acupressure, chiropractic medicine, massage therapy, osteopathy, and reflexology.

Mind/body control explores the mind's ability to affect the body. Therapies include hypnosis, meditation, psychotherapy, support groups, tai chi, and yoga.

Pharmacological and biological treatments involve drugs and vaccines that are not accepted by mainstream medicine. These include anti-oxidizing agents, metabolic therapy, and oxidizing agents.

## Alternative Health Services in the U.S., 2000

Source: *Nutrition Business Journal*

| Health Care Practice | Licensed practitioners | Lay or other practitioners | Total revenues[1] |
|---|---|---|---|
| Acupuncture | 5,800 | 3,000 | $730 |
| Chiropractic | 62,000 | 4,000 | 15,620 |
| Homeopathy | 1,900 | 1,000 | 500 |
| Massage therapy | 38,000 | 150,000 | 7,540 |
| Naturopathy | 21,000 | 2,060 | 3,310 |
| Traditional Oriental medicine | 11,000 | 15,000 | 3,150 |
| **TOTAL** | 139,700 | 175,000 | $30,850 |

(1) In millions of dollars.

## Top-Selling Medicinal Herbs in the U.S., 1998–2000

Source: *Nutrition Business Journal*

| HERB | Sales in 1998[1] | Sales in 1999[1] | Sales in 2000[1] | % change 1998–2000 |
|---|---|---|---|---|
| Echinacea | $208 | $214 | $210 | 1 |
| Garlic[2] | 198 | 176 | 174 | -12 |
| Ginkgo biloba | 300 | 298 | 248 | -17 |
| Ginseng | 217 | 192 | 173 | -20 |
| St. John's wort | 308 | 233 | 170 | -45 |
| Saw palmetto | 105 | 117 | 131 | 25 |
| Combinations | 1,762 | 1,740 | 1,821 | 3 |
| All other | 862 | 1,101 | 1,204 | 40 |
| **TOTAL** | $3,960 | $4,070 | $4,131 | 4 |

(1) In millions of dollars.
(2) Does not include nonmedicinal use.

# Fact and Fiction About Chiropractic[2]

FROM *ALTERNATIVE MEDICINE: A SELECTION OF ARTICLES ON COMPLIMENTARY AND INTEGRATIVE THERAPIES*, MARCH 2002

Relieving low back pain—which affects 80%–90% of American adults at some point in their lives—has become one of modern medicine's holy grails. Even though nine out of ten people recover within a month without any treatment, our society spends more than $20 billion annually on medical care and disability compensation for back pain and injuries.

Despite decades of research, back pain remains as immutable as it is ubiquitous. Chiropractic is a system of treatment that attempts to solve the problem of back pain—and beyond. Practitioners of this century-old method carefully twist, press, or pull on a person's neck, shoulders, back, and hips in an attempt to restore normal motion and relieve pain. Each year, 15 million to 20 million Americans visit chiropractors.

Indeed, nearly everyone knows someone who swears by chiropractic—and not necessarily for back problems alone. Some chiropractors, a vocal minority, assert that manipulating the spine can alleviate such conditions as headache, asthma, and high blood pressure. Critics, on the other hand, counter that such claims remain unproven.

The truth about chiropractic probably lies somewhere in between. Although there is some evidence that spinal manipulation can temporarily relieve low back pain and, to a lesser extent, muscle spasms, strains, or sprains in the neck and shoulders, claims that chiropractic can treat other medical conditions lack scientific support.

## How Chiropractic Began

Chiropractic derives from a Greek word meaning "done by hand." It was born in 1895, when an Iowa grocer named Daniel Palmer allegedly restored the hearing of a nearly deaf man by manipulating his spine. Palmer became convinced that pinched nerves caused by misalignments—or subluxations—of the vertebrae were responsible for almost all diseases. He thought that people would be healed of

---

2. Excerpted from the March 2002 Special Health Report *Alternative Medicine: A Selection of Articles on Complimentary and Integrative Therapies,* © 2002, President and Fellows of Harvard College.

whatever ailed them once their spinal columns were adjusted to the correct position. Fueled by this belief, Palmer and his original supporters eschewed the modern medicine of the day.

Over time, chiropractors split into numerous factions. Some continued to focus solely on manually manipulating the spine to correct the subluxations that they believed triggered disease; others broadened their scope to include nutritional counseling or holistic healing approaches, such as homeopathy and herbal therapy.

*Chiropractic has slowly gained some acceptance from the medical community.*

Chiropractors of another small but growing faction renounce the chiropractic philosophy of subluxation and disease, but believe that there is a legitimate role for spinal manipulation in the treatment of low back pain. The National Association of Chiropractic Medicine (NACM) represents this view.

Because there is no scientific evidence to support the theory on which chiropractic was founded—that most diseases are caused by malfunctioning nerves—medical doctors have traditionally been skeptical of the field. Until 1980, the American Medical Association (AMA) deemed chiropractic an "unscientific cult" and declared it unethical for doctors to refer their patients to chiropractors. That policy changed in 1987 after five chiropractors won an antitrust suit against the AMA in which the medical association was found to have engaged in a conspiracy in restraint of trade.

Since then, chiropractic has slowly gained some acceptance from the medical community, in part, because chiropractors have become more willing to have their treatments evaluated in clinical studies. Today, chiropractors are licensed to practice in all 50 states, and most health insurers cover chiropractic—although, in general, only for back and neck pain.

### Chiropractic in Practice

A landmark event in support of spinal manipulation came in 1994, when the federal Agency for Health Care Policy and Research (AHCPR) issued practice guidelines for treating *acute* low back pain (discomfort lasting less than a month that does not appear to arise from a serious underlying cause). After reviewing more than 4,000 studies on low back pain, an expert panel concluded that spinal manipulation appears to provide temporary relief of acute low back pain.

However, the panelists emphasized that the data support spinal manipulation only when used as a short-term therapy. Whether numerous visits to a chiropractor can provide additional benefit or whether manipulation can reduce the rate of recurrent episodes of back pain remains unknown.

Subsequently, however, in a study published in the *New England Journal of Medicine*, researchers from the University of Washington provided new data that qualified the AHCPR's conclusions. The researchers divided 321 people who had low back pain that had lasted for at least a week into three groups. One group received up to nine visits with a chiropractor; the second had a similar number of session with a physical therapist; and the final group had no special treatment other than an educational booklet on back pain. The people who went to physical therapists learned specific exercises designed to alleviate back pain; those who visited chiropractors underwent spinal manipulation.

While the results did not contradict AHCPR recommendations about chiropractic, they didn't show that undergoing spinal manipulation was any better than performing back exercises. The chiropractic and physical therapy groups recovered at the same rate,

---

### *In general, spinal manipulation appears to be safe for people with uncomplicated back pain.*

---

which was slightly faster than that of the control group. There was no difference among the three groups in terms of missed work, reduced activity, or recurrent episodes of low back pain during the subsequent year.

### Back to Basics

Keeping in mind that 90% of people with acute back pain recover on their own within six weeks, individuals must weigh for themselves whether visiting a chiropractor for short-term relief is worth their time or money. People who feel it works for them should not hesitate to stick with it. However, it's important to see a primary care doctor when back pain interferes with daily activities so he or she can rule out conditions that would require medical attention such as a fracture, infection, or tumor.

In general, spinal manipulation appears to be safe for people with uncomplicated back pain; very few adverse effects have been reported in clinical studies. However, people with rheumatoid arthritis, sciatica (leg pain caused by nerve pressure or damage), and osteoporosis should consult a medical doctor first, because it is possible that spinal manipulation could worsen these conditions.

There is some, although less convincing, research indicating that chiropractic adjustment of the upper back can temporarily ease neck pain. Experts sound a note of caution when it comes to manipulation of the high spine (neck area); this sort of manipulation can worsen an already damaged spinal cord and, in rare cases, compress a neck artery and cause a stroke.

## Choosing a Chiropractor

An individual with low back pain who decides to try chiropractic should ask his or her doctor to recommend a chiropractor with a good track record. Look for one who treats primarily musculoskeletal conditions and who frequently consults with medical doctors. The NACM can also provide referrals.

Although a chiropractor may have reason to take a back x-ray during an initial visit, be skeptical if he or she order such x-rays repeatedly or performs full-spine x-rays, which are believed to be of little diagnostic benefit. Find another chiropractor if you are being pushed to use nutritional supplements or herbal products as part of the therapy. Finally, use common sense. Stop therapy immediately if you feel the adjustments have made the pain significantly worse.

---

### Guidelines for Chiropractic

Here are guidelines from the Agency for Health Care Policy and Research for chiropractic manipulation for the treatment of acute low back pain:

- Chiropractic manipulation can be helpful for patients with acute low back problems (without nerve involvement) when used within the first month of symptoms.
- When findings suggest progressive or severe neurologic defects, appropriate diagnostic assessment to rule out serious neurologic conditions is indicated before beginning manipulation therapy.
- There is sufficient evidence to recommend chiropractic manipulation for patients with spinal nerve problems.
- A trial of chiropractic manipulation in patients without spinal nerve problems is probably safe but effectiveness in unproved.
- If manipulation has not resulted in improvement of symptoms that allows increased functioning after one month of treatment, manipulation should be stopped and patient should be reevaluated.

# Acupuncture³

*MONKEYSHINES ON HEALTH & SCIENCE*, 2002

Acupuncture originated during the ancient times of Chinese healing with the help of natural medicines in 2700 B.C.E. The Chinese Emperor Shen Nung, who used herbs to benefit the health of people, also started the practice of acupuncture.

Acupuncture involves inserting needles, usually a quarter inch to one inch deep, into specific areas of the body to reduce pain and to treat certain disorders.

The art of acupuncture grew from ancient Chinese beliefs from 3000 B.C.E. about what modern medicine classifies as the nervous and circulatory systems. Barefoot Needle Doctors, doctors that practiced acupunture in the rural areas of China, and Chinese physicians believed that when someone became ill the area of pain or problem was out of equilibrium (balance) with the rest of the body.

The use of acupuncture on the areas of the body was believed to support harmony and to restore the correct flow of energy, Qi ("chee"), of the body. The Chinese believed that after acupuncture was performed, the correct amount and balance of energy would return to the body.

Sterilized needles were inserted into the lines (channels) that the Chinese believe run through the body. The Chinese thought that these lines had a direct effect on the patients' energy because they affected the major organs and regions of the body.

Once the needles were inserted, they were twirled and pecked to stimulate (activate) the body to obtain DeQi (the arrival of Qi). The patient may feel tingling or be numb in the areas the needles were put in.

Specific points of pressure and relief have been discovered where acupuncture will benefit the person the most. There are many different types of acupuncture.

The use of heat, or moxibustion, has been added to the needles to promote better blood circulation. Auricular Therapy, ear acupuncture, and scraping, also called Gua Sha are varying forms of the procedure that are used with massage to promote the patient's health.

Acupuncture has been proven to aid patients suffering from a variety of ailments. Treatment can benefit people with muscular and nervous system complications. Sinus problems can be reduced by using acupuncture within the problem area. Disorders of the stomach have also improved in patients who use acupuncture.

---

3. Article from *Monkeyshines on Health & Science* 2002. Copyright © *Monkeyshines on Health & Science*. Reprinted with permission.

The number of treatments a person receives can vary and changes with each individual situation and condition. The type of condition and the patient's reaction to the treatment determines the number of treatments necessary to receive the full benefits of acupuncture.

# A Healthy Balance

## How Homeopathy Helps the Body Heal Itself[4]

By Maria Rabat
*Vegetarian Times*, April 2002

Meghan Malone, a working mother of three, doesn't think she needs to run to the pediatrician for her kids' every sniffle. And frankly, she's wary of antibiotics. When her youngest, Kyle, came home from school with a sore throat, stuffy nose and chills, she gave him a combination homeopathic cold and flu remedy. The next morning, Kyle joined in the usual raucous morning mayhem at the Malone residence. His cold was far from gone, but his symptoms had subsided considerably. By the next day, he was back in school.

Four years ago, Donna Reno's husband dragged her into the office of Todd Rowe, an M.D. trained in psychiatry and a licensed homeopathic physician. Donna didn't put any stock in homeopathy and was almost certain Rowe couldn't do anything for her lupus—an autoimmune disease that attacks the joints, muscles and organs—or her chronic back pain. But nothing else (not even steroids or chemotherapy) had helped. And her husband, Steve, had found that homeopathy relieved his headaches and sinusitis, and he hoped it could ease the constant pain his wife was in.

After an in-depth consultation that covered everything from childhood illnesses and past relationships to Donna's favorite foods and pet peeves, Rowe prescribed a single dose of kali carbonicum, highly diluted potassium carbonate. Within a week, Donna's back pain subsided. Within a month, her lupus symptoms had abated. She hasn't had a flare-up in three years.

These scenarios illustrate the two faces of homeopathic treatment and the possibilities it offers. In classic homeopathy, a practitioner explores a patient's physical, mental and emotional symptoms, then prescribes a single-ingredient remedy. But with today's do-it-yourself drugstore homeopathy, people treat themselves with multi-ingredient "shotgun" remedies, hoping that something in the mix will hit the target and heal them.

### A Kinder, Gentler Medicine

Homeopathic medicine is built on the idea that the body actively seeks balance—physical, mental and emotional—and is capable of self-healing. Its unusual goal is to assist the body's healing energies by producing the same symptoms of illness experienced by a patient,

---

4. Article by Maria Rabat from *Vegetarian Times* April 2002. Copyright © *Vegetarian Times*. Reprinted with permission.

using carefully formulated remedies. In theory, the extra symptoms stimulate the body to correct the imbalance.

Homeopathy is based on three core concepts:

- like cures like (the law of similars)

- the smaller the dose, the more potent it is (the law of infinitesimals)

- the best treatments use a single medicine—and are based on a person's physical and emotional health.

According to the law of similars, substances that cause certain symptoms in healthy people can prod the body to overcome similar symptoms during illness. For example, chopping an onion gives many people a runny nose and watery eyes. Allium cepa, a homeopathic remedy made from red onion, is often prescribed to help fight colds or allergies that have the same drippy, teary symptoms.

Homeopathy's second guiding principle, the law of infinitesimals, states that the more diluted a remedy, the stronger and more lasting its effect. In fact, homeopaths believe the most effective dose is the minimum amount necessary to produce a response.

The third principle—the law of the single remedy—states that the most effective result will come from the one ingredient, given for the least amount of time, that best mimics all of the body's symptoms, physical and emotional.

Americans are increasingly turning to homeopathy because, unlike conventional medicines, they find it convenient, inexpensive and very low-risk. More and more drugstores are stocked with homeopathic treatments for cold, flu and allergies. Yet while classical homeopaths are pleased with their discipline's soaring popularity, many are less than thrilled with the one-size-fits-all approach to what has always been a highly individualized method of healing.

In fact, the multi-ingredient remedies found in drugstores go completely against homeopathic precepts. "Case in point," says Susan Sonz, director of the New York School of Homeopathy in Manhattan, "is a product called Stress Mints, a dual breath freshener and anti-stress remedy. It's a 30C dosage, which means it's quite strong, yet it's a medicine that's marketed as candy," she says. "And that's not all.

## Stocking Your Medicine Cabinet

If you'd like to try homeopathic remedies but don't know where to start, here are 12 remedies that can be used as first aid for common, minor health problems. All are free of animal products.

**Aconite.** (monkshood) for early stages of a cold

**Arnica.** (mountain daisy) for injuries, bruises and muscle soreness

**Belladonna.** (deadly nightshade) for sore throats, earaches and fever

**Calendula.** (marigold) for topical application to cuts, minor burns and diaper rash

**Chamomilla.** (chamomile) for teething, colic and irritability in children; for menstrual cramps

**Cimicifuga.** (black cohosh) for menstrual cramps accompanied by breast soreness

**Cocculus.** (Indian cockle) for motion sickness

**Euphrasia.** (eyebright) for allergies with watery, burning eyes

**Gelsemium.** (yellow jasmine) for flu with body aches; headache

**Nux vomica.** (poison nut) for digestive upsets due to over indulgence in food or alcohol

**Pulsatilla.** (wind flower) for PMS

**Urtica urens.** (stinging nettle) for burns and hives

Mint interferes with homeopathic remedies, which should only be taken when the mouth is free of tastes or flavors."

So as the business of homeopathy continues to boom, how are the Meghan Malones supposed to know which remedies are valid? And just as important, what are we to make of Donna Reno's astounding remission?

### Shaken, Not Stirred

Homeopathic medicines are made mainly from plants, minerals and chemicals, although about 5 percent are from animal sources. In all, there are about 1,500 single homeopathic remedies (pills, creams, ointments and liquid extracts) listed in the Homœopathic Pharmacopœia of the United States, the official compendium.

*Americans are increasingly turning to homeopathy because, unlike conventional medicines, they find it convenient, inexpensive and very low-risk.*

Adhering to the law of infinitesimals, remedies are created through a dilution process called "potentization." The first step is to make an extract from the healing substance. Next, a tincture is created by adding alcohol. Single drops of tincture are repeatedly diluted with water to create the different potencies seen on labels. Common potencies are 6X, 12X and 30X (30 being the most dilute) and 6C, 12C, and 30C ("C" solutions are 100 times more dilute than "X" solutions). But remember that in homeopathy, the smaller the dose—that is, the greater the dilution—the higher the potency. So a 6C remedy is stronger than a 6X, even though the 6C is far more dilute.

An integral part of potentization is the vigorous shaking between each dilution, called succussion. Homeopaths believe that succussion extracts the inherent energy from the healing substance. For instance, if the remedy is made from chamomile, very little to none of the flower may be left in the final dilution. But homeopaths believe that as the remedy becomes less "material" it becomes more "energetic." In theory, each dilution strengthens the remedy and enables it to act in a deeper, more molecular fashion in the body.

### Put to the Test

Until very recently, the medical community has flat out opposed homeopathy. Not surprisingly, dilution—and the shortage of accepted studies proving that it works—has been a huge obstacle scientifically. Lab analysis can't detect any of the original substance in the test material—just water. But these tests do show that on a molecular level, the water has been electromagnetically altered, indicating that there is some type of mechanism at work.

Despite the skepticism, patient support and confidence has kept homeopathy alive. A 1998 report in the *Journal of the American Medical Association* revealed that Americans paid almost 2 million visits to homeopathic practitioners in 1997, a 47 percent increase since 1990. According to Jay Borneman, CEO of the Standard Homeopathic Company and a member of the board of directors for the National Center for Homeopathy (NCH), annual retail sales for homeopathic remedies in the United States are around $300 million and growing at about 8 percent annually. Those are numbers mainstream medicine simply can no longer ignore.

While the latest research is hardly profuse, and results are often open to interpretation, some studies have given homeopathy a much-needed boost. Most of the credible research is being done in Britain, France and Germany, where the medical communities are more open to homeopathy. Two examples:

- A recent study at the Royal London Homeopathic Hospital found that a homeopathic gel (Spiroflor) rubbed onto 161 osteoarthritis sufferers "was as effective and as well-tolerated" as the conventional anti-inflammatory gel, piroxicam (*Rheumatology*, July 2000).

- Almost simultaneously, the *British Medical Journal* published a study of 50 patients with nasal allergies. Half were treated with a 30C preparation, half were given a placebo—and 28 percent of patients in the homeopathic group improved, versus 3 percent in the placebo group.

*Annual retail sales for homeopathic remedies in the United States are around $300 million and growing at about 8 percent annually.*

### The Doctor Is In

Typically, a homeopathy practitioner spends close to two hours on an initial consultation. Not many self-prescribers have the time or training to undergo such a thorough contemplation of the self. And forget grasping the subtleties of the hundreds of homeopathic remedies available! So *is* it possible to self-treat successfully? And do the drugstore remedies work?

Sonz is not a proponent of self-prescribing or of multi-ingredient combo remedies for ailments like colds and flu. "But," she says, "cold and flu remedies have always been lumped together in conventional medicines, and so manufacturers, knowing how important convenience is, are making homeopathic combo remedies for the scads of consumers looking to do something healthy with little effort." However, Sonz adds, "Users will initially experience some benefit, but they will ultimately be giving themselves short shrift by confusing their bodies with multiple remedies, which interrupts the natural healing process. And they may miss out on the deeper, long-term benefits associated with single doses."

But Lorrie Van Overloop, owner of Nature's Market Place in Ridgewood, N.J., gives her customers a bit more credit when it comes to self-prescribing. "Most of them really map out their ailments and have a pretty good idea of what they need. And they buy

---

## Where to Find a Homeopath

While there's a push to establish formal four-year homeopathic medical schools and consistent standards, right now a practitioner's training could be anything from a month-long course to 20 years of study and practice. Only three states—Arizona, Connecticut and Nevada—license medical doctors specializing in homeopathy, and severalaccrediting organizations certify practitioners: the Council on Homeopathic Certification, North American Society of Homeopaths, American Board of Homeotherapeutics, and the Homeopathic Academy of Naturopathic Physicians.

The National Center for Homeopathy puts out a Membership Directory and a Homeopathic Resource Guide, valuable tools for finding a qualified practitioner in your area. Ask around too. Once you've got the names of a few H.P.s, ask how long they've been in practice, what types of training they have, and how experienced they are at treating your problem.

---

single remedies, which suggests that they're aware of the differences between combo and single remedies. Six or seven years ago, they would turn to me for advice. Today, they're much more informed."

### The Fine Print

While homeopathic medicines are not expensive—generally no more than $12—going to a homeopathic practitioner (H.P.) could set you back some. Initial consultations run anywhere from $175 to $250. Many insurance companies will pay for the visit if the H.P. is also a medical doctor (M.D.), an osteopath (D.O.), a naturopath (N.D.) or a chiropractor (D.C.), although there may be more stringent limits on the number of visits or the amount covered.

Moreover, it's foolhardy to rely on homeopathy for all your medical needs. Fractures, surgery and life-threatening illnesses should obviously be handled by specialists. As for Donna Reno's dramatic lupus remission, Sonz admits that that kind of success is experienced by fewer than half of all patients with similar disorders. Finally, while rare, there are reports of adverse reactions to some homeopathic products, ranging from mild rashes to anaphylactic shock—a potentially fatal allergic reaction.

Acute ailments, such as colds, coughs, sore throats, flu, allergies, sinusitis, headaches, sprains and PMS, seem to have the most success with homeopathic treatments. So do your homework. Read labels. Keep an open mind. But if homeopathy does work for you, you'll find you've added an arsenal of gentle, natural remedies to your health care.

# Herbal Medicine: Use with Caution and Respect[5]

BY BRIAN T. SANDEROFF
*GENERATIONS*, WINTER 2000–2001

Throughout history, people have been using plants for medicines. Through a slow process of trial and error, they eventually learned which plant substances could be used to treat which ailments. Written records for Chinese herbal medicine date back over 3,500 years. The first known Chinese book on herbs lists 365 medicinal plants and their uses. Ancient Egyptian texts have described the use of particular plants for treating maladies. Ancient Greek physicians like Hippocrates and Galen laid the foundations of modern Western medicine through herbal medicine. Indeed, even the Bible describes the medicinal use of plants, including the aloe vera plant. Today, a number of herbs are commonly used by older people for medicinal purposes.

The notion that because a substance is "natural" or "comes from nature," it cannot cause harm is false. Arsenic is a substance that occurs naturally yet, when consumed internally, will cause grave illness or death. Various commercial concerns have tried to further the notion that "natural" is equivalent to "safe and effective" which is not true.

Herbal products must be thought of as drugs. Plant substances contain hundreds, sometimes even thousands, of bioactive compounds. Bioflavonoids, flavones, lactones, glycosides, polysaccharides, essential oils, and terpenes are but a few of the types of biologically active substances found in herbs (Agnihorti and Vaidya, 1996; Min et al., 1999; Wu et al., 1991). These sorts of ingredients can affect every kind of function or action within the human body, including enzymatic reactions, receptor-site activation, receptor-site blocking, and protein synthesis (Perry et al., 1998; Nathan, 1999). These effects may be subtle or profound, depending upon a host of factors—the form and concentration of the herb, the part of the plant used, the time period of treatment, even the environment in which the plant was grown or the time of year it was harvested.

In comparison, a pharmaceutical drug is usually a single, isolated chemical compound, for several reasons. First of all, "invented" chemical entities are patentable and thus able to provide a means by which the pharmaceutical company can make

---

5. Reprinted with permission from *Generations*, pg. 69–74, Winter 2000–2001. Copyright © 2001 American Society on Aging, San Francisco, California. *www.asaging.org*.

| Sales of Herbal Remedies in 1998 and 1999 | | | |
|---|---|---|---|
| Herb | 1999 Rank | 1999% of Sales | 1998% of Sales |
| Echinacea | 1 | 7.93 | 9.79 |
| Ginkogo Biloba | 2 | 6.11 | 7.38 |
| St. John's Wort | 3 | 5.46 | 9.10 |
| Garlic | 4 | 4.40 | 6.53 |
| Aloe Vera | 5 | 3.70 | 3.57 |
| Valerian | 6 | 3.33 | 2.30 |
| Kava Kava | 7 | 3.23 | 1.66 |
| Saw Palmetto | 8 | 3.07 | 4.82 |
| Black Cohosh | 9 | 2.84 | N/A |
| Cayene | 10 | 2.80 | 1.76 |

Source: Whole Foods Survey, 1999

money. Second, it is much easier to conduct clinical testing under strictly controlled conditions with a single chemical entity. It is very difficult to perform double-blinded, placebo-controlled, crossover studies with herbs because of the hundreds of active compounds within the herb. It is nearly impossible to standardize all of the ingredients, especially when all of the active compounds have yet to be identified.

Of the number of different compounds within an herb, some may be identified as the active ingredient. Others may be known to contribute to bioavailability, helping the active ingredients get absorbed and delivered within the body. Others may be known to help cut down on side effects (which is a particular problem when dealing with the isolated, individual chemicals found in prescription medicines). Still others may actually be known to cause bothersome but not life-threatening side effects, as is the case with foxglove, and these side effects may warn of overdose before the person's life actually becomes threatened.

Herbs are commercially available in many forms—the dried herb in the form of tea, hydroalcoholic tinctures, capsules and tablets, and poultices, for example. Herbs may be found as single products or in combination with other herbs in a formula for a specific clinical outcome or treatment. Generally speaking, one way to have assurance that the amount of active ingredient within an herbal product is constant from pill to pill and bottle to bottle is to make sure the herbs have been standardized, a process of analysis by which a minimum percentage of an individual ingredient is known to be contained within an amount of the raw herbal material. For instance, hypericin is thought to be the active ingredient within the herb St. John's wort that works as an antidepressant. The typical standardization of hypericin is 0.3 percent. So, a 300 mg capsule of St. John's wort, standardized to 0.3 percent hypericin, will contain at least 0.9 mg of hypericin. Producers assume that if one or two of the important ingredients are standardized, then all of the other ingredients will be standardized as well. However, this assumption is possibly faulty. The concentration of a particular ingredient within an herb can vary for numerous reasons. These include the climate in which an herb is grown, the content of the soil within which the herb is planted, the amount of sunlight the herb is exposed to, the chemicals and pesticides used to treat the herb, and the time of year the herb is harvested. Also, identification of the active ingredient is not always accurate. In the case of St. John's wort, it is now believed that numerous compounds within the herb cause its antidepressant activity, not just the hypericin, as was formerly thought.

*Herbs may . . . interact in positive or negative ways with various prescription medications.*

Herbs may also interact in positive or negative ways with various prescription medications. If an herb and a medication share similar mechanisms of action, the prescription medication may become more effective when the medication is taken with the herb than if it were taken alone, possibly leading to increased risk of toxicity. Conversely, if an herb has a mechanism of action that is in opposition to that of a particular medication, the effect of the drug may be decreased or nullified. Also, some herbs can make the body more efficient at clearing medications from the body, usually by means of mediating liver or kidney function, which can cause the medication to have a decreased physiological effect. Last, some herbs share protein-binding sites (transport mechanisms throughout the body) with certain drugs, thus making more of the drug biologically available and increasing its action within the body.

The concerns mentioned above are not reasons to avoid using herbs. They are, however, very compelling reasons to use herbs with the utmost care and respect, as should be the case with prescription medicines. A qualified healthcare professional who has a working clinical knowledge of both western medicine and herbalism is the best resource for competent advice. This person may be a physician, pharmacist, nurse, chiropractor, or acupuncturist.

This person will not be a physician or pharmacist who has not studied herbalism and who tells the patient that there is no science behind using herbs in response to questions about an herbal remedy. The truth is that there is ample scientific evidence for the medicinal use of hundreds of herbs. But all too often, patients are taking herbal supplements and hiding it from their doctors. They do so because physicians often make their patients fed silly or unintelligent for using herbal supplements, and some patients are of the opinion that their physicians do not know enough about herbal products or have an undue bias against the use of herbal supplements. It is vital for patients to fully disclose the use of herbal products to their physicians. Whether a particular physician is educated about herbal products and how the physician reacts to the idea of patients using herbs should be a determining factor in the patient's choice of a physician.

It is estimated that $3.87 billion is spent annually on herbal products, botanicals, "nutraceuticals" and dietary supplements (Newton et al., 2000). The top ten herbs purchased in the United States from November 1998 to October 1999 are listed in the table on page 158. It is interesting to note that sales of the entire category of herbal supplements increased over the past year, but sales of many of the individual herbs in the top ten actually decreased as a percentage of total sales. This change means that consumers are becoming more interested in a wider variety of herbs available and that they are expanding their repertoire of herbs to use for themselves and their families.

---

*It is estimated that $3.87 billion is spent annually on herbal products, botanicals, "nutraceuticals" and dietary supplements.*

---

Following is a brief discussion about specific herbs that are commonly used by older people.

### Ginko Biloba

Ginkgo biloba is one of the most popular herbs used by older people because of its reported effectiveness in helping to treat memory problems, tinnitus, and Alzheimer's disease and other forms of dementia, among other maladies. The leaves of the ginkgo tree contain many active compounds. Researchers have determined that the whole extract is more active than any of the individual components (much to the chagrin of the pharmaceutical industry). The compounds within the plant have been shown to act as a selective blood platelet aggregation antagonist, a vasodilator, a blood vessel tone regulator, and an antioxidant. The compounds also increase the rate of transmission of information to nerve cells, protect nerve cells as a result of damage from tissue anemia and lack of oxygen, and aid the cells in the use of oxygen and glucose (Clostre, 1999; Fugh-Berman and Cott, 1999).

A 1988 review of twenty different clinical trials, eleven of which were double-blind, estimated that overall efficiency ranged from 44 to 92 percent (Warburton, 1988). Most of the studies used 120 mg of the standardized ginkgo biloba daily, either in one dose or divided into two doses. The conclusions of the researchers were that many categories of older patients could benefit from ginkgo biloba. The data support its use in patients suffering from vascular disorders and dementias and in patients with decreased intellectual function associated with depressed states.

Typically, ginkgo biloba will be standardized to 24 percent flavoglycosides and 6 percent terpened lactones, often referred to as Ginkgo 24/6. Results may take four to six weeks to begin to appear but should continue to accumulate as treatment continues. Some dramatic changes may not appear for up to six months. Side effects are very rare. Ginkgo biloba must be used with caution while being taken with other blood-thinning agents, including Coumadin or aspirin, and patients should always tell their doctors that they are taking ginkgo biloba.

## St. John's Wort

In Europe, St. John's wort is commonly prescribed by physicians for the treatment of depression, just as frequently as the prescription selective serotonin reuptake inhibitors like Prozac (SSRIS). St. John's wort has been reported to help reduce symptoms of mild-to-moderate depression, anxiety, apathy, and insomnia. The flowers and leaves of St. John's wort supply numerous bioactive compounds, including hypericin, and its biological actions have been shown to have several effects in the body, including some similar to those of SSRIS.

Two recent literature reviews show the efficacy of using St. John's wort for depression, although both expressed the need for studies that are better designed (Kim, Streltzer, and Goebert, 1999; Josey and Tackett, 1999). In a 1996 review of twenty-three different studies with 1,757 depressed patients, Linde and colleagues found the hypericin content ingested ranged from 0.4 mg to 2.7 mg daily, usually in a divided dose. The researchers concluded that St. John's wort was superior to placebo in treating some types of depression, but they could not draw firm conclusions about its effectiveness as compared to prescription medicines. St. John's wort did, however, produce fewer side effects than prescription medications.

The most common standardization of St. John's wort is at 0.3 percent hypericin. A 300 mg capsule of the standardized herb will supply 0.9 mg of hypericin, which is then taken in doses of from one to three capsules a day. The time needed to see results can vary from a few days to four to six weeks of daily, consistent use. Mild gastrointestinal disturbances may occur in some patients. Photosensitivity is a reported side effect, but this report stems from observation of cows that graze on wild St. John's wort and consume much more than any human would use therapeutically. St. John's wort may interact with prescription antidepressant medicines, including the MAO inhibitors, SSRIS, or tricyclics, and with the nutritional supplement L-5-HTP, which is a nutritional precursor to serotonin (Lantz, Buchalter, and Giambanco, 1999). St. John's wort should not be taken in conjunction with any prescription medicines without close medical supervision. The Food and Drug Administration advises against taking St. John's wort with any one of 50 other medications, including anticancer agents, heart medications, and drugs for HIV. For a complete list of medications see *www.fda.gov/cder/drug/advisory/stjwort.htm* at the FDA'S website.

### Saw Palmetto

Saw palmetto, a large fan palm shrub that grows in the warm climates of the southern United States, produces a berry that is reported to help alleviate the symptoms of benign prostatic hyperplasia (BPH). In fact, saw palmetto berry extract is a leading treatment for BPH in Germany and Austria. Among the plant's many bioactive components, it is the fatty acids and sterols that have been identified as the most active ingredients.

A 1998 meta analysis of eighteen randomized studies, sixteen of which were double-blind, compared saw palmetto against placebo and Finasteride, a prescription medication for BPH (Wilt et al., 1998). The results were that saw palmetto showed significant improvement in symptom scores when compared to placebo and similar improvement as with Finasteride, but with fewer side effects (such as erectile dysfunction). In a 1994 open trial involving 505 patients with mild to moderate BPH, the results showed significant improvement in symptom scores, urinary flow rates, residual urinary volume, and prostate size after 45 days of treatment (Braeckman, 1994).

The required daily dose of saw palmetto is 320 mg of the liposterolic extract, standardized to contain 85 percent to 95 percent fatty acids and sterols. Side effects are rare, and there are no reports of adverse effects from long-term use. Symptoms often will begin to abate within two weeks, but it may take as long as three months of treatment to see an effect. A proper diagnosis of BPH from a physician is vital before self-treatment of prostatic symptoms with saw palmetto should be undertaken.

### Black Cohosh

Growing in the shady woodlands of the United States and Canada, the roots of the black cohosh plant may provide a safe alternative to synthetic hormones in treating menopause and other female reproductive symptoms, especially for those who cannot use estrogen replacement therapy because of risk of breast cancer. In fact the different chemical entities in black cohosh may inhibit the growth of estrogen-dependent breast cancer cells.

A study by Stolze (1982) involving 704 patients and 131 practitioners looked at the effect of black cohosh on menopausal symptoms. The results were that in 80 percent of the cases, favorable results were obtained including relief of neurovegetative complaints (hot flashes, sweating, headache, vertigo, palpitations, tinnitus) and psychiatric symptoms (nervousness, irritability, depression). The researchers' conclusions were that black cohosh is safe and effective as a hormone-free therapeutic treatment for menopause. A 1987 double-blind study involving 80 patients compared the effects of conjugated estrogens, black cohosh, and placebo on neurovegetative symptoms, anxiety, and proliferation status of vaginal epithelium (Stoll, 1987). The results were that all three areas showed significant improvement with the use of black cohosh when compared to placebo, and the researchers concluded that black cohosh produced safe and efficacious results and is a suitable treatment of choice in menopausal symptoms.

A typical dose of black cohosh would be 40 mg of the herb standardized to 2.5 percent triterpene glycosides taken four times daily. The most common side effect is mild gastrointestinal distress, which is usually relieved by taking black cohosh with food. Other side effects may include dizziness, visual dimness, headaches, tremors, joint pain, and slowed heartbeat. German researchers recommend that treatment be limited to six months. Recent toxicology studies on rats suggest that black cohosh is safe for long-term use, though long-term human studies have not yet been done. Black cohosh should not be taken during pregnancy and may intensify the side effects of oral contraceptives or synthetic estrogens.

## Valerian

The pungent root of the valerian plant, originally from Eastern and Central Europe, has been used to relieve anxiety and chronic or periodic insomnia related to nervousness. Valerian has been shown to depress the central nervous system and reduce smooth muscle spasms.

A 1982 study by Leathwood and colleagues involving 128 volunteers looked at the effect of valerian on sleep quality and sleep latency. At the conclusion of the study, the volunteers reported subjective improvements in ratings for sleep quality and the time it took to fall asleep. Those who had been found to be habitually poor sleepers or those who had taken a long time to fall asleep appeared to have the best results. No "hangover" effect like that which is common with synthetic sedative drugs was reported.

A typical dose of valerian is 150 mg to 300 mg of the extract, standardized to 0.8 percent valerenic acid and 1-1.5 percent valtrates. For insomnia, valerian should be taken thirty to forty-five minutes before bedtime. Consistent administration for two weeks may be needed to see optimal results. There are no common side effects, but on raze occasions an individual may develop a paradoxical reaction of nervousness and excitability. Although German researchers report that it has no interactions with prescription medications, because of possible central-nervous-system depression, it would be wise to use the substance with caution with other medications or substances with a like mechanism of action, including alcohol.

## Conclusion

In conclusion, it is clear that herbs have much in common with prescription medication, including possible powerful effects on the body and the potential for side effects and interactions. Herbs also have a tendency to be more gentle, and more supportive of whole systems and general constitutions in the body, and are much more affordable for the patient—and much less regulated by the United States government. Herbs may be safe and effective for home use, but they should be used in the proper forms and with the advice of qualified health professionals who can offer appropriate guidance.

## References

Agnihorti, S., and Vaidya, A. D. 1996. "A Novel Approach to Study Antibacterial Properties of Volatile Components of Selected Indian Medicinal Herbs." *Indian Journal of Experimental Biology* 34(7): 712–5.

Braeckman, J. 1994. "The Extract of Serenoa Repens in the Treatment of Benign Prostatic Hyperplasia: A Multicenter Open Study." *Current Therapeutic Research* 55: 776–85.

Clostre, F. 1999. "Gingko Biloba Extract (EGb 761). State of Knowledge in the Dawn of the Year 2000." *Annals Pharmaceutiques Francaises* 57(Suppl I): 158–88.

Fugh-Berman, A., and Cott, J. M. 1999. "Dietary Supplements and Natural Products as Psychotherapeutic Agents." *Psychosomatic Medicine* 61(5): 712–28.

Josey, E. S., and Tackett, R. L. 1999. "St. John's Wort: A New Alternative for Depression?" *International Journal of Clinical Pharmacological Therapy* 37(3): 111–9.

Kim, H. L., Streltzer, J., and Goebert, D. 1999. "St. John's Wort for Depression: A Meta-Analysis of Well-Defined Clinical Trials." *Journal of Nervous and Mental Diseases* 187(9): 532–8.

Lantz, M. S., Buchalter, E., and Giambanco, V. 1999. "St. John's Wort and Antidepressant Drug Interaction in the Elderly." *Journal of Geriatric Psychiatry and Neurology* 12(1): 7–10.

Leathwood, P. D., et al. 1982. "Aqueous Extract of Valerian Root (Valeriana Officianalis) Improves Sleep Quality in Man. Reduces Sleep Latency to Fall Asleep in Man." *Pharmacology, Biochemistry and Behavior* 17: 65–71.

Linde, K., et al. 1996. "St. John's Wort for Depression: An Overview and Meta-Analysis of Randomized Clinical Trials." *British Medical Journal* 313: 253–7.

Min, B. S., et al. 1999. "Inhibitory Effect of Triterpenes from Cratagegus Pinatifida on HIV-I Protease" (letter). *Planta Medica* 65(4): 374–5.

Nathan, P. 1999. "The Experimental and Clinical Pharmacology of St. John's Wort (Hypericum Perforatum L.)." *Molecular Psychiatry* 4(4): 333–8.

Newton, G. D., et al. 2000. "New OTC Drugs and Devices 1999: A Selective Review." *Journal of the American Pharmaceutical Association* 40(2): 222–33.

Perry, E. K., et al. 1998. "Medicinal Plants and Alzheimer's Disease: Integrating Ethnobotanical and Contemporary Scientific Evidence." *Journal of Alternative and Complementary Medicine* 4(4): 419–28.

Stoll, W. 1987. "Phytopharmacon Influences Atrophic Vaginal Epithelium: Double Blind Study—Cimicifuga vs. Estrogenic Substances." *Therapeuticum* 1: 23–31.

Stolze, H. 1982. "An Alternative to Treat Menopausal Complaints." *Gynecology* 3: 14–16.

Warburton, D. M. 1988. "Clinical Psychopharmacology of Ginkgo Biloba Extract."

*Gynecology* 3: 327–45.

Wilt, T. J., et al. 1998. "Saw Palmetto Extracts for Treatment of Benign Prostatic Hyperplasia: A Systematic Review." *Journal of the American Medical Association* 280(18): 1604–9.

Wu, J. B., et al. 1991. "Biologically Active Constituents of Centipeda Minima: Sesquiterpenes of Potential Anti-Allergy Activity." *Chemical Pharmacology Bulletin* 30(12): 3272–5.

# Important Health Care Terms

# Important Health Care Terms

**artery:** Blood vessels that carry blood away from the heart. All arteries carry oxygen-rich blood, except the pulmonary artery and its branches, through which oxygen-poor blood is pumped from the heart to the lungs.

**assisted-living community:** A type of living arrangement in which personal care services such as meals, housekeeping, transportation, and assistance with activities of daily living are available as needed to people who still live on their own in a residential facility. In most cases, the "assisted living" residents pay a regular monthly rent. Then, they typically pay additional fees for the services they get.

**blood pressure:** Pressure of the blood against the walls of the blood vessels.

**cancer:** A term for more than 100 diseases in which abnormal cells multiply without control.

**chiropractic:** An alternative medical system. It focuses on the relationship between bodily structure (primarily that of the spine) and function, and how that relationship affects the preservation and restoration of health. Chiropractors use manipulative therapy as an integral treatment tool.

**continuing-care retirement community (CCRC):** A housing community that provides different levels of care based on what each resident needs over time. This is sometimes called "life care" and can range from independent living in an apartment to assisted living to full-time care in a nursing home. Residents move from one setting to another based on their needs but continue to live as part of the community. Care in CCRCs is usually expensive. Generally, CCRCs charge monthly fees and require a large payment before residents move in.

**copayment:** In some Medicare health plans, the amount members pay for each medical service, such as a doctor's visit. A copayment is usually a set amount paid for a service, for example, $5 or $10 for a doctor's visit. Copayments are also used for some hospital outpatient services in the Original Medicare plan.

**deductible:** The amount a patient must pay for health care before the inusrance company or Medicare begins to pay (see **Medicare**). This amount can change every year.

**diaphragm:** The muscle that separates the chest from the abdomen.

**dietary supplements:** A product (other than tobacco) taken by mouth that contains a "dietary ingredient" intended to supplement the diet. Dietary ingredients may include vitamins, minerals, herbs or other botanicals, amino acids, and substances such as enzymes, organ tissues, and metabolites. Dietary supplements come in many forms, including extracts, concentrates, tablets, capsules, gelcaps, liquids, and powders. They have special requirements for labeling. Under DSHEA (Dietary Supplement Health and Education Act), dietary supplements are considered foods, not drugs.

**elder care:** Public, private, formal, and informal programs and support systems, government laws, and ways to meet the needs of the elderly, including housing, home care, pensions, Social Security, long-term care, health insurance, and elder law.

**emphysema:** Chronic lung disease in which there is permanent destruction of the alveoli.

**group health plan:** A health plan that provides health coverage to employees, former employees, and their families, and is supported by an employer or employee organization.

**health care provider:** A person who is trained and licensed to give health care. Also, a place licensed to give health care. Doctors, nurses, hospitals, skilled nursing facilities, some assisted living facilities, and certain kinds of home health agencies are examples of health care providers.

**health maintenance organization (HMO):** A type of Medicare managed care plan where a group of doctors, hospitals, and other health care providers agree to give health care to Medicare beneficiaries for a set amount of money from Medicare every month. In an HMO, members usually must receive all their care from the providers that are part of the plan.

**hemorrhage:** General term for loss of blood caused by injury to the blood vessels or by a low level of the blood elements necessary for clotting.

**HMO with a point of service option (POS):** A managed care plan that lets members use doctors and hospitals outside the plan for an additional cost.

**home health care:** Skilled nursing care and certain other health care available in the home for the treatment of an illness or injury.

**homeopathic medicine:** An alternative medical system. In homeopathic medicine, there is a belief that "like cures like" meaning that small, highly diluted quantities of medicinal substances are given to cure symptoms, when the same substances given at higher or more concentrated doses would actually cause those symptoms.

**hospice:** Hospice is a special way of caring for people who are terminally ill, and for their family. This care includes physical care and counseling. Hospice care is covered under Medicare Part A (Hospital Insurance). See **Medicare**.

**hypertension:** High blood pressure.

**long-term care:** A "variety" of services that help people with health or personal needs and activities of daily living over a period of time. Long-term care can be provided at home, in the community, or in various types of facilities, including nursing homes and assisted living facilties. Most long-term care is custodial care. Medicare does not pay for this type of care.

**mammogram:** A special x-ray of the breasts. Medicare covers the cost of a mammogram once every 12 months for women over 40 who are enrolled in Medicare.

**Medicaid:** A joint federal and state program that helps with medical costs for some people with low incomes and limited resources. Medicaid programs vary from state to state, but most health care costs are covered if individuals qualify for both Medicare and Medicaid.

**Medicare:** The federal health insurance program for people 65 years of age or older, certain younger people with disabilities, and people with End-Stage Renal Disease (permanent kidney failure with dialysis or a transplant, sometimes called ESRD).

Individuals are eligible for premium-free (no cost) Medicare Part A (Hospital Insurance) if:

• They are 65 or older and are receiving, or are eligible for, retirement benefits from Social Security or the Railroad Retirement Board, or

• They are under 65 and have received Railroad Retirement disability benefits for the prescribed time and meet the Social Security Act disability requirements, or they or their spouse had Medicare-covered government employment, or

• They are under 65 and have End-Stage Renal Disease (ESRD).

If they are not eligible for premium-free Medicare Part A, they can buy Part A by paying a monthly premium if:

• They are age 65 or older, and

• They are enrolled in Part B, and

• They are residents of the United States and are either citizens or aliens lawfully admitted for permanent residence who have lived in the United States continuously during the 5 years immediately before the month in which they apply.

Individuals are automatically eligible for Part B if they are eligible for premium-free Part A. They are also eligible for Part B if they are not eligible for premium-free Part A, but are age 65 or older *and* residents of the United States, citizens, or aliens lawfully admitted for permanent residence. In this case, they must have lived in the United States continuously during the 5 years immediately before the month during which they enroll in Part B.

**Medicare private fee-for-service plan:** A private insurance plan that accepts people with Medicare. Individuals may go to any Medicare-approved doctor or hospital that accepts the plan's payment. The insurance plan, rather than the Medicare program, decides how much it will pay and what patients will pay for the services they receive. They may pay more for Medicare-covered benefits. They may also have extra benefits the Original Medicare Plan does not cover.

**Medicare supplement insurance:** Medicare supplement insurance is a Medigap policy. It is sold by private insurance companies to fill "gaps" in Original Medicare Plan coverage. Except in Minnesota, Massachusetts, and Wisconsin, there are 10 standardized policies labeled Plan A through Plan J. Medigap policies only work with the Original Medicare Plan. See also **Medicare**.

**network:** A group of doctors, hospitals, pharmacies, and other health care experts hired by a health plan to take care of its members.

**nursing home:** A residence that provides a room, meals, and help with activities of daily living and recreation. Generally, nursing home residents have physical or mental problems that keep them from living on their own. They usually require daily assistance.

**preferred-provider organization (PPO):** A managed care in which members use doctors, hospitals, and providers that belong to the network. They may use doctors, hospitals, and providers outside of the network for an additional cost.

**premium:** The periodic payment to Medicare, an insurance company, or a health care plan for health care coverage.

**primary care:** A basic level of care usually given by doctors who work with general and family medicine, internal medicine (internists), pregnant women (obstetricians), and children (pediatricians). A nurse practitioner (NP)—a State licensed registered nurse with special training—can also provide this basic level of health care.

**pulmonary artery:** Blood vessel that delivers oxygen-poor blood from the right ventricle of the heart to the lungs.

**red blood cells:** Cells that transport oxygen from the lungs to all tissues of the body.

**referral:** Permission from a primary care doctor for a patient to see a specialist or obtain certain services. In many Medicare managed care plans, members need a referral before they receive care from anyone except a primary care doctor. If a member does not get a referral first, the plan may not pay for care.

**respite care:** Temporary or periodic care provided in a nursing home, assisted living residence, or other type of long-term care program so that the usual caregiver can rest or take some time off.

**squamous cell carcinoma:** Cancer that begins in the flat scale-like cells in the skin and in tissues that line certain organs of the body including the larynx.

**stem cells:** Primitive cells that are the building blocks of all other cells in the human body. Because stem cells can develop into specific kinds of cells, from them, researchers can grow specialized cells or tissue, which could be used to treat injuries or disease. Stem cell research is controversial because the best source of stem cells is human fetal tissue harvested from an embryo that will be destroyed in the process.

**trachea:** Airway that connects the larynx to the lungs; also called the windpipe.

# Bibliography

# Books

American Psychiatric Association. *Diagnostic and Statistical Manual of Mental Disorders: DSM-IV*. 4th ed. Washington D.C.: American Psychiatric Association, 1994.

Andersen, Ronald M., Thomas H. Rice, and Gerald F. Kominski, eds. *Changing the U.S. Health Care System: Key Issues in Health Services, Policy, and Management*. San Francisco: Jossey-Bass, 1996.

Black, Kenneth Jr., and Harold D. Skipper Jr. *Life & Health Insurance*. 13th ed. Upper Saddle River, NJ: Prentice Hall, 2000.

Burke, Mary M. *Primary Care of the Older Adult: A Multidisciplinary Approach*. St. Louis: Mosby, 2000.

Cichoke, Anthony J. *Secrets of Native American Herbal Remedies*. New York: Avery Penguin Putnam, 2001.

Evans, Timothy, et al., eds. *Challenging Inequities in Health: From Ethics to Action*. New York: Oxford University Press, 2001.

Hankinson, Susan E., et al., eds. *Healthy Women, Healthy Lives: A Guide to Preventing Disease from the Landmark Nurses' Health Study*. New York: Simon & Schuster Source, 2001.

Jennings, Marian C., ed. *Health Care Strategy for Uncertain Times*. San Francisco: Jossey-Bass, 2000.

Khalsa, Dharma Singh, and Cameron Stauth. *Meditation As Medicine: Activate the Power of Your Natural Healing Force*. New York: Pocket Books, 2001.

Lebow, Grace, Barbara Kane, and Irwin Lebow. *Coping with Your Difficult Older Parent: A Guide for Stressed-Out Children*. New York: Avon Books, 1999.

Litman, Theodor J., and Leonard S. Robins. *Health Politics and Policy*. 3rd ed. Albany: Delmar Publishers, 1997.

Loverde, Joy. *The Complete Eldercare Planner*. 1st ed. New York: Hyperion, 1997.

McDonough, John E. *Experiencing Politics: A Legislator's Stories of Government and Health Care*. Berkeley: University of California Press, 2000.

National Academy of Sciences. *Crossing the Quality Chasm: A New Health System for the 21st Century*. Washington, D.C.: National Academy Press, 2001.

Northrup, Christiane. *The Wisdom of Menopause: Creating Physical and Emotional Health and Healing during the Change*. New York: Bantam Books, 2001.

Northrup, Christiane. *Women's Bodies, Women's Wisdom: Creating Physical and Emotional Health and Healing*. Rev. ed. New York: Bantam Books, 1998.

Powell, Francis D., and Albert F. Wessen, eds. *Health Care Systems in Transition: An International Perspective*. Thousand Oaks, CA: Sage Publications, 1999.

Shapiro, Molly. *HMOs and the Patient's Bill of Rights*. Freedom, CA: Crossing Press, 1999.

Shortell, Stephen M., et al. *Remaking Health Care in America: The Evolution of Organized Delivery Systems*. San Francisco: Jossey-Bass, 2000.

Sinatra, Stephen, Jan DeMarco Sinatra, and Roberta Jo Lieberman. *Heart Sense for Women: Know the Real Risks of Heart Disease in Women and Design Your Total Plan for Natural Prevention and Treatment*. Washington, D.C.: LifeLine Press, 2000.

Sultz, Harry A., and Kristina M. Young. *Health Care USA: Understanding its Organization and Delivery*. 3rd ed. Gaithersburg, MD: Aspen Publishers, 2001.

# Web Sites

This section offers the reader a list of Web sites that can provide more extensive information on specific diseases and ailments, preventive techniques, treatment options, and ways to donate time and money to specific causes. These Web sites also include links to other sites that may be of help or interest. Due to the nature of the Internet, the continued existence of a site is never guaranteed, but at the time of this book's publication, all of these Internet addresses were in operation.

**Alzheimer's Association** *www.alz.org*

**American Cancer Society** *www.cancer.org*

**American Diabetes Association** *www.diabetes.org*

**American Parkinson's Disease Association** *www.apdaparkinson.com*

**Arthritis Foundation** *www.arthritis.org*

**Lupus Foundation of America** *www.lupus.org*

**National Headache Foundation** *www.headaches.org*

**National Multiple Sclerosis Society** *www.nmss.org*

**National Osteoporosis Foundation** *www.nof.org*

**National Stroke Association** *www.stroke.org*

**National Cancer Institute** *www.cancer.gov*

## Other Web Sites

### American Heart Association
*www.americanheart.org*
Describes different heart conditions and posts facts, research, and treatment options for heart disease and heart attacks.

### American Liver Foundation
*www.liverfoundation.org*
Provides information, preventive strategies, and treatment options for hepatitis and other liver diseases.

### American Lung Association
*www.lungusa.org*
Promotes the fight against lung disease while placing an emphasis on environmental health, asthma, and tobacco control.

### The Center for Medicare and Medicaid Services
*www.hcfa.gov*
Provides information on medicare and medicaid.

## Centers for Disease Control and Prevention (CDC)

*www.cdc.gov*
Government agency and devoted to research into preventing and controlling all types of diseases.

## Centers for Disease Control, Divisions of HIV/AIDS Prevention

*www.cdc.gov/nchstp/hiv_aids/dhap.htm*
Division of the Center for Disease Control focusing primarily on educating and preventing HIV/AIDS, sexually transmitted diseases (STDs), and tuberculosis (TB).

## JAMA (Journal of the American Medical Association)

*www.jama.ama-assn.org*
Provides articles, editorial letters, and book reviews on different medical topics affecting the public at large. It also conducts debates on controversial issues, discusses medical trends, and provides a news source that benefits medical professionals as well as nonmedical-affiliated readers.

## Mayo Clinic

*www.mayohealth.org*
Provides information on a variety of current health questions and concerns.

## Medicare Info

*www.medicare.gov*
Geered towards people with medicare. Provides answers to frequently asked questions, provides a list of participating physicians, and outlines coverage and other useful information for those with medicare.

## The National Heart, Lung and Blood Institute

*www.nhlbi.nih.gov*
Provides information on the causes, preventive measures, diagnoses, and treatments of heart, blood vessel, lung, and blood disease, as well as sleeping disorders.

## National Institutes of Health

*www.nih.gov*
Provides information on this official government medical research center.

## National Kidney Foundation

*www.kidney.org*
Provides information on different forms of kidney disease, organ donations, transplants, and educational activities for the afflicted and their families.

## Women's Health

*www.womens-health.org*
Provides information on this not-for-profit agency dedicated to research in an attempt to improve women's health.

# Additional Periodical Articles with Abstracts

More information on health care can be found in the following articles. Readers who require a more comprehensive selection are advised to consult *Readers Guide to Periodical Literature, Readers Guide to Abstracts, Social Science Abstracts*, and other H.W. Wilson publications.

**Your Aging Parents: How to Help.** Nuna Alberts. *American Health*, v. 14 pp54–7+ April 1995.

Alberts reports that more than 80 percent of elder care comes from family members or people who live with the older person, according to social scientist Katrina Johnson. These caregivers sometimes pay a toll physically and emotionally because of their responsibilities. Nevertheless, caring for an elderly relative can be a rewarding experience if everyone's expectations are made clear from the start. The article discusses how to get the proper diagnosis for an elder's problems, the shortage of doctors trained in geriatrics, how caregivers can get help and information, determining whether home care is appropriate, and relief for stressed caregivers.

**Medical Mayhem.** Monique R. Brown. *Black Enterprise*, v. 32 pp102–9 August 2001.

Brown writes that, as doctors, employers, and insurance providers fight over health care issues, patients are caught in the cross fire. Most Americans are members of employer-sponsored managed health care programs. Under such schemes, insurance providers pay doctors a predetermined sum for each patient under their care. The benefits of the system are that doctors are guaranteed payment, as well as a stream of patients from the plan's enrollees, and that health care costs are contained. Now that the cap is coming off health care costs, however, employers are predicting that premiums will rise by 8 percent to 20 percent in 2002. Rising costs in the pharmaceutical industry are adding further pressure. The benefits of managed care are not as apparent to doctors or their patients: Doctors resent intrusion into medical decisions by insurance companies, and patients want to choose their doctors and have a say in treatment options.

**Securing the Golden Years.** Linda Marsa. *Black Enterprise*, v. 19 pp62–6+ December 1988.

Marsa explains how proper planning by both children and their elderly parents can make the parents' retirement years more rewarding. Planning should begin before the parents retire so that they may utilize any special perks in their employee benefit packages. The first step is to talk openly about money while being sensitive to the parents' changing position of authority, security, and control within the family. Seek financial advice from experts who specialize in geriatrics, or contact a local aging office or senior-citizens' group for information on free seminars on postretirement planning. Successful planning strategies are described, and sources of additional information are listed.

**Biotech for Boomers.** Catharine Arnst. *Business Week*, pp152–5 August 20–27, 2001.

Arnst writes that new treatments will become available in the next few years to help some patients manage once-deadly diseases. The writer discusses new biotechnological developments that will help baby boomers manage cancer, Alzheimer's, and heart disease.

**Arresting Alzheimer's.** Naomi Freundlich. *Business Week*, pp94–6 June 11, 2001.

Freundlich reports that drugs that fight milder memory loss may prevent the onset of Alzheimer's disease. By the time victims develop Alzheimer's, their brains are usually too damaged for any treatment to do much good. So drug companies are increasingly turning their attention to a different type of patient—one who suffers from noticeable memory loss but otherwise functions normally. The theory is that treating patients with this condition, called mild cognitive impairment, could delay or deter full-blown Alzheimer's. New drugs in the pipeline aim to either boost the brain's ability to form memories, despite the buildup of brain-clogging plaque formed by an insoluble protein called beta-amyloid, or slow the plaque buildup.

**Be Wary of Health Discount Cards.** *Consumer Reports*, v. 67 pp8–9 May 2002.

The magazine describes how medical discount cards have pitfalls of which consumers may not be aware. Holders of these cards pay a monthly fee in the range of $10 to $120, depending on the plan, and are promised reduced rates at participating pharmacies, hospitals, and dentists' and doctors' offices when the card is presented. Discount card schemes are not regulated in most states, and the people who sell the cards are not obliged to be licensed or have any health care experience. Moreover, being able to decipher whether the holder is getting a true discount is difficult because detailed price lists from participating providers are not usually available or verifiable. There is also no control over how companies use the confidential medical information supplied when the card is used for treatment. Ultimately, the programs are not a replacement for health insurance.

**Sports-Supplement Dangers.** *Consumer Reports*, v. 66 pp40–2 June 2001.

The magazine reports that some sports-supplement products supposedly increase muscle or energy but could cause serious harm. Americans spent around $1.4 billion on sports supplements in 1999, hoping the pills, drinks, and powders would help them put on weight, slim down, or compete better. The few good scientific studies available on these "dietary" supplements indicate that they either are ineffective or, at best, produce only small changes in performance. More disturbing, they can contain potent and potentially harmful substances, such as androstenedione, which can upset the body's hormonal balance when it metabolizes into testosterone and estrogen and may cause premature puberty and stunted growth in adolescents. Consumers merely have to enter a food-supplement store to get these products, says Gary Wadler, a New York sports-medicine specialist and adviser to the White House Office of National Drug Control Policy.

**Who Gets Health Care?** Robert W. Fogel and Chulhee Lee. *Daedalus*, v. 131 pp107–17 Winter 2002.

The writers say that concern is growing internationally about who receives health care. Numerous studies demonstrate that the differences in various measures of health between the affluent and the poor remain wide, despite the long-term tendency toward a healthier society. Some researchers contend that the gulf is actually widening. They suggest that this may be due to a shift in the health care system in advanced industrial countries from the basis of universal access to a more market-oriented system; increasing income disparity is another possible cause. The writers discuss what constitutes an "essential" health care system and the optimal combination of private and government contributions to health care services.

**Environment and Health: Issues for the New U.S. Administration.** Kirk R. Smith. *Environment*, v. 43 pp34–42 May 2001.

According to Smith, a major factor driving concerns about environmental quality is its connection to human health. Health has been at the root of much of the environmental research, legislation, and control efforts undertaken around the world in recent decades. Although it is quite clear how important health is in the environment arena, it is less clear how important the environment is in the health arena. People's knowledge of the current and potential future determinants of human health is discussed.

**Don't Harden Your Heart.** Donald D. Hensrud. *Fortune*, v. 144 pp254 September 3, 2001.

Hensrud explains how in May, National Institutes of Health (NIH) experts urged Americans to get tough on high cholesterol. If the NIH recommendations are followed, there could be a 25 percent increase in the number of people on cholesterol-reducing drugs and a large decrease in fatalities from heart disease, the top killer in the United States. Low-density lipoprotein cholesterol is unfavorable because it travels from the liver to the artery wall, increasing plaque buildup, like an old pipe slowly clogging. High-density lipoprotein cholesterol is beneficial because it does the opposite, taking plaque from the artery wall back to the liver and out of the body. LDL cholesterol can be lowered through diet, and HDL cholesterol can be increased by exercising, losing weight, and giving up smoking.

**The Traitor Within.** Louise Jarvis. *Harper's Bazaar*, pp150–6 February 2001.

According to Jarvis, strange symptoms, difficult detection, and no known cure are making autoimmune disease a major women's health problem. The disease, a group of 80 noncommunicable illnesses, is currently the fifth-leading cause of death among women aged 15 to 44. One American in five, 75 to 90 percent of whom are women, suffers from at least one of these diseases—lupus, rheumatoid arthritis, multiple sclerosis, Grave's disease, and type 1 diabetes, for example—which develop when the immune system attacks a part of the body as though it were an infection. Autoimmune disease is to the technological age what cancer was to the industrial age, a worrying public health threat whose cause and cure are still elusive.

**New Answers to Menopause?** Timothy Gower. *Health*, v. 16 pp76–82 January/February 2002.

Gower reports that, with continuing doubts about hormone-replacement therapy (HRT), women are seeking natural remedies for menopausal symptoms. The American Heart Association announced in July 2000 that it did not recommend HRT as an intervention to prevent heart attacks and that there is insufficient evidence that restoring a woman's hormone levels protects her heart. According to a federally funded study of women from the age of 45, more than 20 percent of subjects used only alternative approaches to cope with menopausal symptoms, and 25 percent used both traditional and alternative treatments. The writer discusses soy, black cohosh, red clover, evening-primrose oil, and dong quai as alternatives to HRT.

**Out of the Shadows.** Jane Bennett Clark. *Kiplinger's Personal Finance*, v. 55 pp88–92 January 2001.

Clark writes that depression affects over 19 million adults in America and racks up more than $43 billion per year in medical costs, lost productivity, and absenteeism. Although most people with depression stay in the workforce, the disease can complicate other medical conditions and lead to permanent disability. Advances in research have rendered mental illnesses much more treatable than in the past, however. People with major depression usually respond well to talk therapy and medication. Bipolar disorder is considered harder to treat, but it can usually be managed with therapy and drugs. The growing effectiveness of drug therapy and Ashland, Virginia–based attorney William Herbert's struggle with depression are among the topics discussed.

**Between Home and Nursing Home.** Mary Beth Franklin. *Kiplinger's Personal Finance*, v. 54 pp72–6 September 2000.

Franklin explains that over the last two decades, assisted living has gained a reputation as a good alternative to nursing-home care for the elderly. In theory, assisted living provides frail elderly people with a place where they can live in a homelike environment while receiving help with all their daily requirements. Opinions are very divided about how well this goal is being achieved, however, with some critics stating that they promise care they are unable to deliver in understaffed facilities. The writer outlines several people's experiences of assisted living facilities, and a sidebar provides information on choosing a suitable home.

**Military Muscle.** Kimberly Lankford. *Kiplinger's Personal Finance*, v. 56 pp120–4 May 2002.

Lankford discusses fitness boot camps, a booming exercise trend in which tough trainers use military methods to get their troops fit. Roughly half of boot-camp recruits have grown bored with weight machines, treadmills, and gym classes that do not work, and, according to former Navy fitness instructor Patrick Avon, even though they have been in aerobics class for years, they are still too heavy. Avon has been running the Sergeant's Program, one of the first fitness boot camps, since 1989; over the past 13 years, he has hired a staff of equally rugged instructors and now works with over 1,000 recruits at about 40 programs in Washington, D.C., and four in Chicago.

**A Season of Discontent.** Leslie Haggin Geary. *Money*, v. 31 pp129–30 April 2002.

Geary offers tips on managing health insurance and controlling bills through low-cost treatments, tax write-offs, using language that an insurer understands, and being aware of employee-assistance-program caveats.

**Challenge of the New Century: Finding an AIDS Vaccine.** David Baltimore. *New Perspectives Quarterly*, v. 18 pp47–9 Winter 2001.

Baltimore writes that the right way to globally eradicate HIV/AIDS would be through vaccination of the population. In the United States, about 10 percent of the annual budget of $2 billion spent on AIDS research goes toward the development of a vaccine. Researchers are still far from finding a vaccine, but two recent experiments have provided hope that it is possible to make a human vaccine for AIDS. One experiment was based on pure DNA injected into monkeys, and if a pure DNA vaccine is developed, it will be safe, cheap, and easy to use everywhere. The other equally hopeful experiment was conducted by Bruce Walker at Boston's Master General Hospital, but it requires close medical surveillance of patients that is not always possible for a whole society, and even less so across an entire continent.

**Searching for a New and Improved Prozac.** Geoffrey Cowley. *Newsweek*, v. 139 pp100–1 December 31, 2001/January 7, 2002.

Cowley explains how drug companies are striving to develop a new and improved Prozac. Prozac and similar medications take weeks to relieve depression; their side effects can range from indigestion to sexual dysfunction; and none of them helps more than two in three patients. Given the fact that depression might be the result not of low serotonin levels but of the atrophy of particular brain cells, drug companies are looking to create pills that offer cleaner, more direct ways of maintaining cells.

**The Skin-Cancer Scare.** Geoffrey Cowley. *Newsweek*, v. 137 pp58 January 29, 2001.

Cowley reports that skin cancer is on the increase in the United States. Occurrences of all three of the major skin cancers—basal-cell carcinoma (BCC), squamous-cell carcinoma, and malignant melinoma—have risen in recent decades as people have spent more free time outside without the proper protection from the sun. There are now almost 1 million cases of BCCs each year, and the numbers of malignant melanomas have increased more than twofold. The writer discusses the nature of the three skin cancers and the risk factors involved.

**Companies Trim Health Benefits for Many Retirees As Costs Surge.** Milt Freudenheim. *New York Times*, ppA1+ May 10, 2002.

Freundenheim writes that, as reflected in this year's annual reports to shareholders, corporate profit earnings have been reduced because of the surging inflation in medical costs. Employers are responding by cutting health benefits or requiring retirees to pay more for coverage. The reductions in benefits stem mainly from increases in the cost of prescription drugs, which account for 40 to 60 percent of retirees' health care. According to the U.S. Chamber of Commerce, health care costs will soar 18 percent this year and future costs are estimated to rise as much as 34 percent.

**Many Doctors Shun Patients with Medicare.** Robert Pear. *New York Times*, pp1+ March 17, 2002.

Pear examines how significant numbers of physicians are refusing to take new Medicare patients. They assert that the government pays too little to cover the costs of treating the elderly.

**Gene Therapy Is on the Horizon.** Bill Sardi. *Nutrition Science News*, v. 6 p386 October 2001.

Sardi considers how the nutrient-envrionment side of the nuture-versus-nature debate is making history. Although the debate continues over whether it is nature in the form of genes, or a combination of diet, environment, and lifestyle that is largely responsible for health and longevity, nutrient-deficiency diseases have been largely eradicated in developed countries. Death from tuberculosis, scarlet fever, measles, and whooping cough have declined as advances in agriculture and transportation make a variety of nutritious foods available. It is questionable whether gene therapy will ever help the poor and infirm to the extent that nutrition can. Ruth Hubbard at Harvard University says that although human genome mapping is heroic, most deaths the world over occur because of a lack of nutritious food, clean water, sanitation, and other inexpensive medications in sufficient levels, rather than bad genes.

**Discover the Healing Power of Chinese Medicine.** Sara Altshul O'Donnell. *Prevention*, v. 51 pp104–11 March 1999.

O'Donnell writes that Chinese medicine, which predates modern medicine by over 2,000 years, has attracted the attention of Western researchers, who are discovering that Chinese therapies are amazingly effective, particularly for women. From fibroids to hot flashes, and more serious illnesses, there is proof that this ancient healing art may have something to offer patients that they cannot get elsewhere. Traditional Chinese Medicine (TCM) practitioners believe that physical symptoms result from an underlying imbalance, and this what they try to mend. TCM treatments are discussed, and the experiences of a number of women are described.

**How to Quit the Holistic Way.** Marianne Apostolides. *Psychology Today*, v. 29 pp35–43+ September/October 1996.

According to Apostolides, holistic therapies are helping to span the gap between conventional, exclusively abstinence-oriented approaches to addiction and the newer, more controversial philosophy of harm reduction. In dealing with an addiction, all holistic techniques start from the premise that people develop addictions to correct an "imbalance" within themselves. Holistic therapies seek to reestablish balance by linking mind and body. They remove some of the fundamental causes of abuse by helping people to become aware of and take responsibility for the way they think, feel, and act. The holistic philosophy overlaps with the harm-reduction approach to addiction, which does not demand that people remain abstinent. It works from the premise that people cannot be compelled to deal with a problem and that people who are treated with respect and who are educated about their choices often choose to help themselves. Massage, hatha yoga, nutrition therapy, acupuncture, hypnosis, and homeopathy are discussed.

**How to Cure Health Care.** Milton Friedman. *Public Interest*, pp3–30 Winter 2001.

The renowned economist explains how medical savings accounts provide one way of resolving the increasing financial and administrative problems associated with Medicare and Medicaid. A medical savings account allows individuals to deposit tax-free funds in an account that can be used only for medical health bills, as long as they have a high-deductible insurance policy that restricts the maximum out-of-pocket costs. The introduction of such accounts would eliminate the problem of those who at the moment are without medical insurance, get rid of the bulk of the bureaucratic structure, free medical practitioners from an ever more onerous burden of paperwork and regulation, and prompt numerous employers and workers to turn employer-provided medical care into higher cash wages. The taxpayer would save money because overall government costs would be dramatically reduced, and the family would no longer face the possibility of a big medical disaster.

**Moving Away from Cancer.** Carol Krucoff. *Saturday Evening Post*, v. 272 pp16+ November/December 2000.

According to Krucoff, exercise, well known to help protect against America's leading killer, heart disease, is increasingly being examined as a potential weapon against the second-highest killer, cancer. The majority of experts concur that regular exercise can cut the risk of colon cancer, and there is increasing agreement that it could also reduce the risk of breast cancer. For those with cancer, there is a growing number of exercise programs available, mainly to help alleviate unpleasant side effects of the disease and its treatments and to boost the overall quality of life. Moreover, there is some indication that physical activity could decelerate the course of the disease. The writer discusses two new studies, presented at the recent annual meeting of the American College of Sports Medicine in Indianapolis, that seem to show that men with high fitness levels are less likely to die of cancer.

**What's a Guy to Do?** Christine Gorman. *Time*, v. 159 pp98 Mar 18, 2002.

Gorman reports that questions have been raised about whether the standard blood test to screen for prostate cancer does more harm than good. Advocates of the prostate-specific antigen test argue that the fall in the death rate from prostate cancer throughout North America since the mid-1990s is a result of the screening that started in the 1980s. According to a study in a recent *Canadian*

*Medical Association Journal*, however, there was no statistical link between screening and death rates in relation to the disease.

**Been Down So Long.** Sanjay Gupta. *Time*, v. 159 pp148 January 21, 2002.

The writer considers whether the couch is still needed for the treatment of depression. Prozac and other new drugs sparked a revolution in the treatment of depression. The downside, however, is that many people are not getting another important treatment for depression: face-to-face therapy. The dangers, critics claim, is that pills are thrown at problems by psychiatrists instead of psychiatrists grappling with the underlying causes.

**The New Science of Alzheimer's.** J. Madeleine Nash. *Time*, v. 156 pp50–7 July 17, 2000.

Nash writes that, as the immense World Alzheimer Congress in Washington draws researchers from around the world, a sense that scientists could be on the brink of halting the epidemic is dawning. Over the past few years, information and astonishing insights into Alzheimer's have begun to emerge from corporate, government, and university laboratories. In addition, due to the influx of interest and research dollars, the pace of discovery is picking up. The writer discusses the history of the disease, while diagrams show how it develops in the brain. Sidebars provide details on scientists researching the disease to determine whether there is a genetic test to detect the disease, and some of its most well-known victims are featured.

**Sport Medicine: To Heal or to Win?** Philippe Liotard. *UNESCO Courier*, v. 53 pp37–9 September 2000.

Liotard explains why advances that have been made in life sciences and biotechnology are raising serious issues for doctors involved in sport medicine. In their relationships with their patients, doctors are trying to reconcile ethical considerations with the new demands arising from a liberal society that highly values efficiency, output, and performance, reflected particularly in the arena of drug-taking in sport. Although doping is generally considered to be unethical in light of an imaginary sporting ideal, this view skims over the real issue of the pressures of competition in sport and masks it even further from the public, doctors, and authorities. Ultimately, the real ethical debate is a question of medical practice that raises the issues of how doctors should respond to requests for drugs from athletes at all levels. The writer discusses how it can be decided when medical interventions actually become efforts to improve performance and outlines how doctors can opt out of the controversy.

**Healthcare Headaches.** Lynn Rosellini. *U.S. News & World Report*, v. 132 pp52–3 April 15, 2002.

According to Rosellini, underinsured students could find out the hard way that the details count. Accustomed to depending on their parents' insurance, many do not read the fine print on the policies offered by schools they are considering or even buy insurance once they have enrolled. Many graduate students still harbor youthful illusions of invulnerability and they gamble that they will not become ill.

Each year, however, many other students lose the gamble and find themselves underinsured, facing huge medical bills.

**The Coming Age of Ecological Medicine.** Kenny Ausubel. *Utne Reader*, pp56–61 May/June 2001.

Ausubel reports that a new understanding of health and illness has emerged that is starting to move away from treating only the individual. Good health depends on the realization that every person is part of a wider web of life, which needs to be healthy for humans to be healthy. One step toward achieving a healthier future lies in ecological medicine, which is a loosely shared philosophy based on advancing public health by improving the environment. Its central thesis is that industrial civilization has made a fundamental mistake in acting as if humans are separate from nature, and the ecological approach to healing borrows from the insights of indigenous healing traditions, including the fact that nature has an extraordinary and mysterious capacity for self-repair. Some basic tenets of ecological medicine are discussed.

**Good Germs, Bad Germs.** Tinker Ready. *Utne Reader*, pp26–8 November/December 2001.

Ready writes that in the June issue of British environmental journal *The Ecologist Report*, Gary Hamilton argues that in the rush to stamp out infectious disease, people could be creating new health threats by interfering with the microbe-laden ecosystems in human bodies and the environment. Hamilton notes that people see how germs make them sick but not how they keep humanity healthy. Instead of thinking of all germs as bad, certain scientists are examining the symbiotic relationships between the human body and various bacteria, fungi, viruses, and protozoa. There is a great deal to learn about how the body is able to tolerate and even benefit from these live-in microbes.

**Health Care Past and Present.** Richard F. Corlin. *Vital Speeches of the Day*, v. 68 pp301–5 Mar 1, 2002.

In an address before the Economic Club of Greater Lansing, Kellogg Center, Michigan State University, the president of the American Medical Association discusses the coming crisis in the health care industry. The speaker notes that health insurance premiums are increasing dramatically, small businesses are making drastic cuts to benefits, and the recession has increased the number of people who are unemployed and without health insurance. He further states that the public health system is attempting to prepare for biological attacks at the same time as state and federal funding is drying up, that U.S. doctors and patients appear to have no safe harbor, and that liability costs are increasing significantly nationwide. Finally, he points out that Congress has reduced reimbursement from Medicare by 5.4 percent and is threatening access to medical care for seniors.

**Science Fiction.** Chris Mooney. *Washington Monthly*, v. 34 pp31–7 April 2002.

Mooney examines how the American public's fascination with complementary and alternative medicine (CAM) has boomed in recent years, and so has the medical community's interest in understanding it. Hundreds of researchers at dozens of medical schools are studying the previously untested techniques, including meditation, acupuncture, herbalism, chelation, colonics, and leech therapy, with the goal of determining which treatments have legitimate medical value and which are mere superstition. This should be good news: Mainstream medicine can assimilate whatever proves worthy, and practitioners of legitimate CAM techniques can finally gain the authority of scientific approval and respect after decades of ridicule. However, the simple fact that medical schools are taking CAM seriously has lent it an air of legitimacy, and in many cases practitioners are deliberately trying to undermine conclusive testing demonstrating the lack of merit in their techniques.

**The Patients' Right Not to Sue.** James D. Miller. *Weekly Standard*, v. 6 pp13–14 August 13, 2001.

Miller argues that congressional sponsors of the patients' bill of rights currently heading for a House-Senate conference want to force everyone to pay higher health insurance premiums in return for the ability to sue. There are individuals who do not want the ability to sue health insurance companies: If an insurance provider knows there is a chance it can be sued, it might charge higher premiums. What is more, there are those who believe that the legal system is an ineffective means for resolving disputes between patients and health insurance companies. They should not be forced to pay higher premiums. If Congress really cared about the rights of patients, Miller contends it would make the patients' bill of rights voluntary.

# Index

Abbott, Randall, 50, 53
actinic cheilitis, 20
actinic keratoses, 20
acupuncture, 144, 150–151
African Americans
    high blood pressure and, 75
    risk of dying from prostate cancer, 16
Agency for Health Care Policy and
    Research (AHCPR), 147, 149
aging and health. *See* elder care
air pollution and lung cancer, 14
alcohol
    heart disease risk factors and, 83
    residential treatment programs. *See*
        detoxification programs
ALFA (Assisted Living Federation of
    America), 107
Alix, Joan, 99–102
Alleger, Irene, 118–119
ALS (amyotrophic lateral sclerosis), 121
alternative medicine
    acupuncture, 144, 150–151
    as remedy for menopause symptoms,
      97
    coverage by health insurers, 5–6
    fields of practice, 143–144
    herbal remedies. *See* herbal remedies
    homeopathy. *See* homeopathy
    prevalence of use worldwide, 143
    types available in U.S., 144
Alzheimer's disease
    care facilities, 111–112
    communication and cuing tips, 113
    fitness professionals' role, 113
    incidence in U.S., 111
    pathology, 108, 110
    rank as cause of death, 107
    stages, 110
    syndrome description, 108
    warning signs, 109
    *See also* elder care

American Medical Association (AMA),
    147
amyotrophic lateral sclerosis (ALS), 121
angina, 7
angiography, 7
anorexia nervosa. *See* eating disorders
antidepressant therapies, 29
antioxidants, 19
antiperspirants and breast cancer myths,
    90
artery, 169
asbestos and lung cancer, 13
aspirin use and heart health, 85
Assisted Living Federation of America
    (ALFA), 107
assisted-living communities, 112, 169
    *See also* nursing homes
Association of Chiropractic Medicine
    (NACM), 147
auricular therapy, 150
autoimmune diseases, 122
Avorn, Jerry, 117

back pain, 146–149
Bailey, Amos, 129, 131, 132–134, 137
Balanced Budget Act (1997), 36
balloon angioplasty, 10
Balm of Gilead, 127–128, 129, 131, 137
Banks, Mark, 52
basal cell carcinoma, 18
BCBS Blue Card Program, 49
Begley, Sharon, 120–122
Benevento, Barbara, 48, 51
benign prostatic hyperplasia (BPH), 162
Benko, Laura B., 42–46
Berardo, Joseph, 49
Berg, Alfred O., 27, 28
Berlin, Michelle, 72
Beyar, Rafael, 122
Bierbower, Beth, 48, 53
Bierman, Arlene, 116
biotechnology
    stem cell research
        federal prohibitions on, 120
        regenerative medicine, 121